CAMBRIDGE LIBRARY COLLECTION

Books of enduring scholarly value

History of Medicine

It is sobering to realise that as recently as the year in which On the Origin of Species was published, learned opinion was that diseases such as typhus and cholera were spread by a 'miasma', and suggestions that doctors should wash their hands before examining patients were greeted with mockery by the profession. The Cambridge Library Collection reissues milestone publications in the history of Western medicine as well as studies of other medical traditions. Its coverage ranges from Galen on anatomical procedures to Florence Nightingale's common-sense advice to nurses, and includes early research into genetics and mental health, colonial reports on tropical diseases, documents on public health and military medicine, and publications on spa culture and medicinal plants.

The Life of Edward Jenner

Active in fields spanning medicine, ornithology, zoology and even water-colour painting, Frederick Dawtrey Drewitt (1848–1942) was a prominent fellow of the Royal College of Physicians, exhibited at the Royal Academy, and was involved in governing the National Trust. His particular interest in birds led him to study the work of the physician and naturalist Edward Jenner (1749–1823), who contributed to the field of ornithology through his observations of the cuckoo's behaviour. Jenner is better known, however, as the 'father of immunology' for pioneering the smallpox vaccination – the word 'vaccine' comes from the Latin *vacca* (cow) as Jenner used the cowpox virus to inoculate against smallpox infection in humans. Drewitt had general readers in mind when he wrote about Jenner's extraordinary life and growing worldwide recognition. The first edition of this biography was published in 1931, and this enlarged second edition appeared in 1933.

T0188083

Cambridge University Press has long been a pioneer in the reissuing of out-of-print titles from its own backlist, producing digital reprints of books that are still sought after by scholars and students but could not be reprinted economically using traditional technology. The Cambridge Library Collection extends this activity to a wider range of books which are still of importance to researchers and professionals, either for the source material they contain, or as landmarks in the history of their academic discipline.

Drawing from the world-renowned collections in the Cambridge University Library and other partner libraries, and guided by the advice of experts in each subject area, Cambridge University Press is using state-of-the-art scanning machines in its own Printing House to capture the content of each book selected for inclusion. The files are processed to give a consistently clear, crisp image, and the books finished to the high quality standard for which the Press is recognised around the world. The latest print-on-demand technology ensures that the books will remain available indefinitely, and that orders for single or multiple copies can quickly be supplied.

The Cambridge Library Collection brings back to life books of enduring scholarly value (including out-of-copyright works originally issued by other publishers) across a wide range of disciplines in the humanities and social sciences and in science and technology.

The Life of Edward Jenner

Naturalist, and Discoverer of Vaccination

F. DAWTRY DREWITT

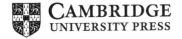
CAMBRIDGE
UNIVERSITY PRESS

CAMBRIDGE UNIVERSITY PRESS

Cambridge, New York, Melbourne, Madrid, Cape Town,
Singapore, São Paolo, Delhi, Mexico City

Published in the United States of America by Cambridge University Press, New York

www.cambridge.org
Information on this title: www.cambridge.org/9781108063487

© in this compilation Cambridge University Press 2013

This edition first published 1933
This digitally printed version 2013

ISBN 978-1-108-06348-7 Paperback

THE LIFE OF
EDWARD JENNER

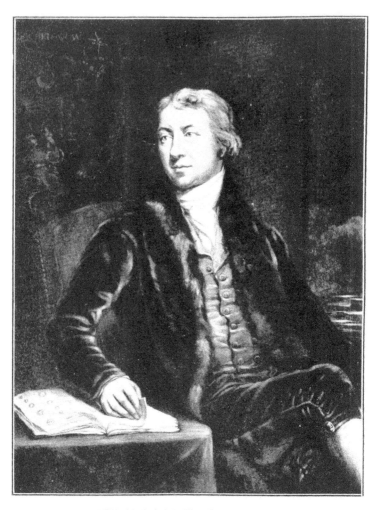

EDWARD JENNER, M.D., F.R.S.

From a mezzotint by W. Say, in the British Museum ; after a portrait by J. Northcote painted for the Medical Society of Plymouth, 1802.

THE LIFE OF
EDWARD JENNER

M.D., F.R.S.

NATURALIST, AND DISCOVERER
OF VACCINATION

BY

F. DAWTREY DREWITT

M.A., M.D., F.R.C.P.

AUTHOR OF 'THE ROMANCE OF THE APOTHECARIES'
GARDEN,' 'BOMBAY IN THE DAYS OF GEORGE IV,'
'LATIN NAMES OF COMMON PLANTS, THEIR
HISTORY, AND PRONUNCIATION'

SECOND EDITION
(ENLARGED)

WITH PORTRAITS AND ILLUSTRATIONS

LONGMANS, GREEN AND CO.
LONDON • NEW YORK • TORONTO
1933

LONGMANS, GREEN AND CO. LTD.
39 PATERNOSTER ROW, LONDON, E.C. 4
6 OLD COURT HOUSE STREET, CALCUTTA
53 NICOL ROAD, BOMBAY
36A MOUNT ROAD, MADRAS

LONGMANS, GREEN AND CO.
55 FIFTH AVENUE, NEW YORK
221 EAST 20TH STREET, CHICAGO
88 TREMONT STREET, BOSTON

LONGMANS, GREEN AND CO.
128–132 UNIVERSITY AVENUE, TORONTO

Made in Great Britain

PREFACE TO SECOND EDITION

' THE Life of Edward Jenner,' by John Baron, was published nearly a century ago. Few of the present generation can have read it; but all naturalists remember his name as the discoverer of the extraordinary activities of the young cuckoo ; and all nations gratefully acknowledge their debt to the man who almost banished smallpox from the earth.

A manuscript notebook kept by him, containing his classical observations on the cuckoo, has been lately published by the Royal College of Physicians. The present writer was requested to contribute an introduction to *Jenner's Note Book*, and was thereby led to the writing of this short account of Jenner's life, in the hope that it may interest some who are neither doctors nor naturalists.

CONTENTS

vii

CONTENTS

LIST OF ILLUSTRATIONS

LIFE OF EDWARD JENNER

CHAPTER 1

Edward Jenner's family. School. Pupil of John Hunter. Refuses post of naturalist on Captain Cook's second voyage. Declines partnership with John Hunter. Returns as country doctor to Berkeley. William Cobbett's description of Vale of Gloucester. Berkeley Castle.

EDWARD JENNER was born on May 17, 1749, at Berkeley, in Gloucestershire—an ideal spot for one destined to be a devoted lover of the English countryside.

The little old town, standing on a gentle eminence, with its feudal castle, overlooked the rich pasture lands of the Vale of Berkeley and the river Severn, where, after long wandering, its waters widen as they near the sea.

Edward was the third son of the Rev. Stephen Jenner, vicar of Berkeley. His mother was a daughter of the Rev. Henry Head, sometime prebendary of Bristol. He was scarcely five when he lost his father ; but the boy was brought up with ' affectionate care and judicious guidance ' by his eldest brother, the Rev. Stephen Jenner, who now succeeded his father at Berkeley.

B

Another brother, the Rev. Henry Jenner, became rector of Rockhampton and vicar of Little Bedwin in Wiltshire. Two sons of this brother (the Rev. George C. Jenner and Henry Jenner) qualified as medical practitioners, and assisted their uncle Edward in his natural history studies and medical practice.

When eight years old Edward was sent to the Grammar School at Wotton-under-Edge, and, later, to a school under the Rev. Dr. Washbourn at Cirencester.

The lad's taste for natural history began to show itself early. Before he was nine he had made a collection of dormice nests, and, while at Cirencester, a much-prized collection of fossils from the oolite. Later on, while still a schoolboy, he studied pharmacy and surgery under Ludlow, a well-known surgeon at Sodbury, near Bristol. Then for two years he was one of John Hunter's pupils in London.

Apprenticeship to a surgeon was at that time the beginning of a medical student's training—an important part of his education. Always in touch with his master, an eager pupil would continually absorb useful knowledge not to be found in books, nor to be learnt in a hospital ward.

Jenner was at that time twenty years of age ; Hunter forty-one, surgeon to St. George's Hospital, and owner of a menagerie at Brompton, where he studied the habits and life-history of animals. 'Penetrating and original thinker,' indefatigable in his search for scientific truth, Hunter was Jenner's hero. Tutor and pupil became friends for life.

In 1771, Captain Cook returned from his successful voyage to the 'Great Southern Continent.' Sir Joseph Banks—afterwards the well-known President of the Royal Society—had furnished Cook's ship. He had provided an artist and a botanist for the expedition, and had brought back a cargo of natural history treasures, including a mass of new plants dried and pressed. They had been collected near the sea, at a spot afterwards named Botany Bay.

Jenner was asked to prepare and arrange all Banks's specimens. This he did with such skill and care that he was offered the appointment of naturalist to Cook's next expedition—to sail in 1772. At the same time Hunter suggested a partnership, as he wished to increase the number of his lectures on comparative anatomy and surgery.

But Jenner had few of the common ambitions of men. These, and other offers, which other men would have proudly accepted, were declined. Jenner preferred to return to the sweet air of his native village[1] to live among country people and

---

[1] Jenner in his letters also talks of the little town of Berkeley as a ' village.'

country creatures, ride along the well-known lanes, and accept the drudgery of a country doctor's life. Like Virgil,[1] he loved rivers and woods more than glory. What for him was the good of ambitious struggling all for the bubble reputation ?

> '. . . What is its reward ?   At best a name.
> Praise—when the ear has grown too dull to hear.
> Gold—where the senses it should please are dead.
> Wreaths—where the hair they cover has grown grey.
> Fame—when the heart it should have thrilled is numb.'[2]

The unexpected — paradoxical — result of this refusal of all likely to lead to fame was that Jenner became famous in all civilised (and in many un-civilised) countries throughout the world.

As a rule, no doubt, Wendell Holmes is right in saying that people gain by being transplanted into new surroundings.   Like trees, they grow more freely on fresh soil.   But for one of Jenner's tempera-ment his was a wise decision, and, as it happened, a fortunate one for the world.   Jenner loved the Vale of Berkeley ; there he found friendliness and understanding between all classes ; and an escape from the smoky air of London, which, he said, choked him.

Above all, it saved him from learning that in-difference to neighbours—that necessary but un-

---

[1] ' *Flumina amem silvasque inglorius.*'   Virgil, *Georg.* ii. line 486.
[2] N. P. Willis.

attractive hardness, which comes to all who have to struggle every day in a crowd—often against women and children.

And it was a beautiful bit of old England to which Jenner returned—the sister Vales of Berkeley and Gloucester. Even half a century later, when agricultural depression and the decay of the countryside had begun, William Cobbett described that corner of England with enthusiasm.

Cobbett was then taking his *Rural Rides*, and pouring out indignation and lamentation at the over-taxation of the land which followed the Napoleonic wars—the ruin of the country yeomen —the poverty of the labourers, and the wealth of war-profiteers, with their harsh manners and ignorance of country ways.

One of Cobbett's journeys was to Gloucester. He writes of the misery of country-folk in and around Marlborough, of the new park at Savernake, where ' 50 to 100 farms of former days ' had been ' swallowed up.' [1]   He rides by ' Cititer ' (Cirencester) through desolate country. ' Anything quite so cheerless ' he does ' not recollect to have seen.' [2]

' This miserable country,' he writes, ' continued to the distance of ten miles, when all of a sudden I looked down from the top of a high hill into the *Vale of Gloucester* ! Never there was, surely, such a contrast in this world !

[1] *Rural Rides*, Nov. 6, 1821.   [2] *Ibid.*, Nov. 8, 1821.

The hill is called *Burlip Hill* ; it is much about a mile down it . . . From this hill you see the Morvan Hills in Wales . . . All here is fine ; fine farms ; fine pastures ; all inclosed fields ; all divided by hedges. Gloucester is a fine, clean, beautiful place ; and, which is of a vast deal more importance, the labourers' dwellings, as I came along, looked good. The labourers themselves pretty well as to health and cleanliness. The girls at work in the fields (always my standard) are not in rags, with bits of shoes tied on their feet, and rags tied round their ankles, as they had in Wiltshire.'

No wonder Jenner loved that country ! Here his kindness, his dexterity as a surgeon, and his modesty with all his accomplishments, seem to have made him a most popular practitioner. He is described as having the ' generosity of a good man, the simplicity of a great one.'

For a time he lived in the Vicarage with the brother to whom he owed his early training. He then took a small house—Chantry Cottage—near the church—laid out the garden with care—planted shrubs and trees—and, later on, kept ' tame pheasants, sheldrakes, and other birds ' in it, as well as an eagle, sent from Newfoundland.

Near by was the great castle—home of the Lords of Berkeley continuously from Norman times. Its owners had taken their share in all the rough life of the Middle Ages, in the old French campaigns, and in the chronic warfare in their own country.

A Lord Berkeley, together with other barons, had fought against the King at Evesham.

When King Edward II, handsome and athletic, but foolish, frivolous and extravagant, and with no set purpose in life, had plunged England into civil war, the third Lord Berkeley was imprisoned in the spacious Roman castle at Pevensey. Queen Isabella, with her son Edward and the baron Mortimer, then raised the country against the King. Lord Berkeley was released.

On returning to his castle Lord Berkeley replenished his manors, and lived in state. Three hundred persons, according to the Berkeley archives,[1] dined every day at the castle. No manor had fewer than 300 sheep ; some had as many as 1500 ; and 15,380 horses were employed. Every farm had its pigeon-house, and 1300 young pigeons were sent every year to the castle. There were ' falcons ' (female peregrines), ' tiercels ' (male peregrines) and ' other hawks ' (goshawks and merlins) which required five or six hens as food every day.

Fox-hunting—at night, with nets and dogs—was Lord Berkeley's favourite and necessary sport, for foxes were numerous and destructive.

Edward II, who had been made a prisoner, was sent to Berkeley Castle, and there, in the absence of the owner, brutally murdered.

---

[1] John Smyth's *Berkeley MSS.*, 1567–1640.

When not fighting, the Lords of Berkeley seem to have been devoted to the cultivation of their pleasant lands. They had a ship, and they exported wool and corn. The fifth Lord Berkeley (so the archives state) was ' a perfect Cotswold sheppard, living a kind of grazier's life, having his flocks of sheep somering in one place, and wintering in another.'

Henry, Lord Berkeley, with his mother and a hundred and fifty servants, attended the Court of Henry VIII—lived in Kentish Town—hunted with hawk and hound in Gray's Inn Fields, Islington, and 'Heygate': then returned to Berkeley—entertained in the castle—sitting ' when neighbours feasted in his hall,' at the bottom of the table, or opposite the salt, between his guests of ' higher or meaner degree.'

Later on, during his absence, Queen Elizabeth visited the castle, and took part in a great slaughter of his herd of red deer. In one day alone twenty-six were killed, others wounded, and the destruction continued. It could not have been a pleasant sight ; for the deer must have been driven together into a net, to provide the Queen and her courtiers with an easy target for their crossbows.

Lord Berkeley was distressed, and threatened to disforest his park. On hearing this—so the books say—the Queen sent him an angry message. But the Berkeley archives tell a different story. A friend at Court warned him to be careful of his words, as ' the Earl (Leicester) had purposely caused that slaughter of his deere,' and ' might have a further plot against his head, and that castle, whereto he had taken no small likinge.'

But the covetous Leicester did not get his way. The Castle remained with the Berkeleys, who, in the eighteenth century, gave valuable help to Jenner in his vaccination campaign.

Jenner must have enjoyed the beauty of the grand building. In his *Note Book*, lately published by the Royal College of Physicians, he mentions the house-martins' nests on its walls—recalling Shakespeare's description of the martins' nests on Macbeth's castle as Duncan enters:

> ' This guest of summer,
> The temple-haunting martlet, does approve,
> By his loved mansionry, that the heaven's breath
> Smells wooingly here : no jutty, frieze,
> Buttress, nor coign of vantage, but this bird
> Hath made his pendant bed and procreant cradle :
> Where they most breed and haunt, I have observed,
> The air is delicate.'

When castles, and churches, and houses of stone appeared in England, the martins left the rocks and chalk cliffs on which they had built their nests, and became *house*-martins—friends of man's household.

Now, man stretches fine wires on his buildings, perplexing house-martins as black threads stretched over beds of flowering crocus perplex house-sparrows. The house-sparrows, too,—parasites of man and enemies of martins—which have driven house-martins from London,[1] increase in number ; so the house-martins are everywhere giving up their right to their newly acquired name, and are leaving man to find other, less pleasant, means of keeping down his flies and mosquitoes.

[1] A well-known ornithologist, the late Mr. Howard Saunders, told the writer that he remembered seeing martins' nests on some houses in Bayswater, but that the birds were driven away by London sparrows.

CHAPTER 2

IN 1773, Jenner began medical practice in a
county he knew well. His family had long been
small landowners there. He shared the house of
his elder brother, and another brother, two sisters,
and an aunt lived near by.

Strong and active, rather under middle height,
in a broad-brimmed hat, blue coat with brass
buttons, and high, well-polished boots, he enjoyed
his long rides through the Vales of Berkeley and
Gloucester and over the Cotswold hills—drinking
in the beauty of the surrounding country. From a
spot named Barrow Hill—a peninsula in a bend of
the river, from whence there were distant views of
the valleys of the Forest of Dean and the Bristol
Channel—Jenner loved to watch the sunset with
sympathetic friends ; and he formed a small club,

the members of which met and dined near by three or four times a year. The scenery, the trees, the flowers, the birds, were a constant delight to him.

Fond of his fellow-creatures, and they of him. Baron describes how his neighbours would accompany him for twenty or thirty miles in a morning, to enjoy his conversation whether ' mirthful or grave. . . . His knowledge and dexterity as a surgeon, his manners as a gentleman, and his general information rendered his company always acceptable. . . . He not only commanded confidence by his skill, but also secured to himself goodwill and affection by the tenderness, kindness, and benevolence of his nature.' [1]

Although Jenner's practice was rapidly increasing, he found time to join a small musical Club, where he occasionally played the violin. He also took a chief part in forming a society for the improvement of medical science, and for the promotion of good fellowship among fellow-practitioners. It met at Rodborough. He was also a member of another medical society which met at Alveston, near Bristol.

As did others of his time, Jenner occasionally indulged in writing light verse. To a lady, who inquired after a patient, he wrote :

' I've dispatched, my dear madam, this scrap of a letter
To say that the patient is very much better.

[1] Baron : *Life of Edward Jenner*, i. 13.

A regular Doctor no longer she lacks,
And therefore I've sent her a couple of Quacks.'

He had sent his patient two ducks. There is a poem of his to a robin which begins :

> ' Come sweetest of the feather'd throng,
> And soothe me with thy plaintive song :
> Come to my cot devoid of fear ;
> No danger shall await thee here,
> No prowling cat——'

His lines on ' Signs of Rain ' show him to be an observant field-naturalist :

> ' The hollow winds begin to blow,
> The clouds look black, the glass is low,
> The soot falls down, the spaniels sleep,
> And spiders from their cobwebs creep.
> Last night the sun went pale to bed.
> The moon in halos hid her head.
> The boding shepherd heaves a sigh,
> For see ! a rainbow spans the sky.
> The walls are damp, the ditches smell,
> Clos'd is the pink-ey'd pimpernel.
> Hark ! how the chairs and tables crack :
> Old Betty's joints are on the rack.
> Loud quack the ducks, the peacocks cry,
> The distant hills are looking nigh.
> How restless are the snorting swine !
> The busy flies disturb the kine.
> Low o'er the grass the swallow wings :
> The cricket too, how loud it sings.

Puss on the hearth with velvet paws
Sits smoothing o'er her whiskered jaws.
Through the clear stream the fishes rise,
And nimbly catch the incautious flies.
The sheep were seen, at early light,
Cropping the meads with eager bite.
Though June, the air is cold and chill ;
The mellow blackbird's voice is still.
The glow-worms, numerous and bright,
Illumed the dewy dell last night.
At dusk the squalid toad was seen
Hopping, crawling, o'er the green.
The frog has lost his yellow vest,
And in a dingy suit is dress'd.
The leech disturbed is newly risen
Quite to the summit of his prison.
The whirling winds the dust obeys,
And in the rapid eddy plays.
My dog, so altered is his taste,
Quits mutton bones on grass to feast ;
And see yon rooks, how odd their flight,
They imitate the gliding kite.
Or seem precipitate to fall,
As if they felt the piercing ball.
'Twill surely rain—I see with sorrow,
Our jaunt must be put off to-morrow.'

Could any official ' forecast ' be more convincing ?

An old-fashioned fair was held at Berkeley every year, to the delight of children for miles round. There were stalls for toys ; and the shows included Jenner's natural history collection. Purchases for

the year were made at such fairs, for there were no
railways to take village folk to the great towns.
Everybody bought something.   It recalls a pretty
old song :

> ' Oh dear ! what can the matter be !
> Johnnie's so long at the fair.
> He promised to buy me a bunch of blue ribbons,
> To tie up my bonnie brown hair.
> He promised . . .'

Jenner describes the fair on a day when there
was no sign of rain :

> ' The sun drove off the twilight gray,
> And promised all a cloudless day ;
> His yellow beams glanced o'er the dews,
> And changed to gems their pearly hues,
> The song birds met on every spray,
> And sang as if they knew the day ;
> The blackbird piped his mellow note ;
> The goldfinch strained his downy throat ;
> The little wren, too, left her nest,
> And, striving, sang her very best ;
> The robin wisely kept away,
> His song too plaintive for the day—
> 'Twas *Berkeley Fair*, and nature's smile
> Spread joy around for many a mile.
> The rosy milkmaid quits her pail ;
> The thresher now puts by his flail ;
> His fleecy charge and hazel crook,
> By the rude shepherd are forsook ;

The woodman, too, the day to keep,
Leaves Echo undisturbed in sleep ;
Labour is o'er—his rugged chain
Lies rusting on the grassy plain.'

The sights of the fair are described, and at the
end of the day

'. . . the clamours die away,
The sun has sent a farewell ray :
The hills have lost their golden hue,
And wrapped themselves in mantle blue ;
The lions all begin to dose,
The tigers seek a soft repose ;
The customer no more is courted ;
And every standing is deserted :
The Fair is o'er.   But joys like these
Long revel in a heart at ease.
The milkmaid, as she skims her cream,
Long on the happy time will dream ;
And many a simple rustic swain
Will strive to whistle out the strain,
While raking up the new-mown hay
All in the merry month of May.
And little girls, and little boys,
Will for a moment quit their toys,
And cling about their mothers' knee,
Asking when Fair again will be ;
And every breast with hope will burn
To see the happy day return.'

It was a pleasant village life to which Jenner
returned.

Then came a change. Jenner, always sensitive,

lost his good spirits. There had been some un-happy love affair. After a time he confides in Hunter, who writes a characteristic letter of condolence : [1]

' Dear Jenner,—I own that I was at a loss to account for your silence, and I was sorry at the cause . . . I can easily conceive how you must feel, for you have two passions to cope with, viz. that of being disappointed in love ; and that of being defeated ; but both will wear out, perhaps the first soonest . . . I want you to get a hedgehog, in the beginning of winter, and weigh him ; put him in your garden, and let him have leaves, hay, and straw to cover himself with, which he will do ; then weigh him in the Spring and see what he has lost.

Ever yours,
JOHN HUNTER.

' 25 Sept. 1778.'

The pang of disappointed love lay heavily on Jenner for many a long year ; but he threw him-self into his work. One day he was summoned to Gloucester Infirmary—a sixteen-mile ride—to operate on an inmate, and had the satisfaction of saving his patient.

A country doctor's life in those days required physical strength and endurance. Jenner describes a ride through a blizzard on the Cotswolds :

' I was under the necessity of going to Kingscote. The air felt more intensely cold than I ever remember to have

---

[1] The letter is in the library of the Royal College of Surgeons.

experienced it. The ground was deeply covered with snow, and it blew quite a hurricane, accompanied with continual snow. Being well-clothed, I did not find the cold make much impression on me till I ascended the hills, and then I began to feel myself benumbed. There was no possibility of keeping the snow from drifting under my hat, so that half of my face, and my neck was for a long time wrapt in ice. There was no retreating, and I had still two miles to go . . . over the highest downs in the country.

' As the sense of external cold increased, the heat about the stomach seemed to increase. I had the same sensations as if I had drank a considerable quantity of wine or brandy ; and my spirits rose in proportion to this sensation. I felt . . . as one intoxicated, and could not forbear singing. My hands at last grew painful, and this distressed my spirits in some degree.

' When I came to the house I was unable to dismount without assistance. I was almost senseless, but I had just recollection enough to prevent the servants from bringing me to a fire. I was carried to the stable first, and from thence was gradually introduced to a warmer atmosphere. I could bear no greater heat than that of the stable for some time. Rubbing my hands in snow took off the pain. My horse lost part of the cuticle and hair from neck and ears. I had not the least inclination to take wine, or refreshment. One man perished a few miles from Kingscote at the same time, and from the same cause.'

Happily, tired wayfarers who take their last long sleep in a snowdrift seem to suffer little pain. Possibly the increased amount of oxygen inhaled with each breath in the cold air was the cause of the exhilaration Jenner felt.

In 1783 the great hall at Berkeley Castle was put to unaccustomed use. That year a French papermaker, Joseph Montgolfier, had made a large 'football,' a 'ballon,' out of packing-cloth and paper—had filled it with hot air from a chafer, and had succeeded in getting it to rise more than 1000 feet into the sky.

Such was the excitement in Paris that a subscription was at once raised to allow Professor Charles of Paris to repeat the experiment. Charles ordered a 'ballon' to be made of varnished silk and to be filled with hydrogen gas. Then, with all the city looking on, in drenching rain, he liberated it from the Champ de Mars. It rose to a height of 3000 feet, descended fifteen miles away, and was attacked and torn to pieces by frightened peasants. The world was intensely interested. The experiment seemed to open up for mankind a prospect of drifting through the air like gossamer spiders.

In order to show Berkeley folk Montgolfier's experiment, Jenner constructed a balloon in the hall of Berkeley Castle, filled it with hydrogen, and, surrounded by wondering neighbours, set it free in the Vale. It sailed over the hills, came down some miles away, and was filled again at Kingscote for another voyage.

That year his nephew, Henry Jenner, became his ' apprentice ' and helped him in his practice.

Jenner was not satisfied with the old belief that all illnesses are due to inflammation, and he worked hard at examining animals, slaughtered for food, in order to trace the beginnings of sickness. His *Note Book*[1] shows the perseverance with which he examined the bodies of diseased animals. Hydatid tumours and tubercle were of such frequent occurrence, that he believed them to be due to the same cause. The extraordinary life-history of the creatures which form hydatid tumours was then unknown, and there was no microscope powerful enough to show the bacilli of tubercle. It was unfortunate that such unpleasant work should have led Jenner along a blind road.

In one of his papers he points out the relation between heart-disease and rheumatism, and recommends that the heart should be ' covered ' in cases of acute rheumatism.

During an epidemic of ophthalmia he writes to the Rev. Dr. Worthington recommending the use of nitrate of mercury ointment, and counter-irri-

[1] The Harveian Librarian to the Royal College of Physicians—Arnold Chaplin, M.D., F.R.C.P.—reports in his Preface to the recently published *Note Book of Edward Jenner*, that the MS. came into the possession of the College in 1888. The book is well printed, and contains an admirable reproduction, by Emery Walker, of Jenner's portrait by Sir Thomas Lawrence, in the Royal College of Physicians.

tation on the temples for the worst cases—both sound treatment. He says :

' In cases of the most violent kind, and which quickly threaten to destroy the eye, I introduce a seton in the temple, about an inch from the outward angle of the eye. The latter practice has, I believe, given sight to thousands since I first made it public, about 1783.'

In 1788 John Hunter's prophecy at last came true. Jenner married Miss Catherine Kingscote, one of a family well known in that part of the country. ' In her counsel and sympathy he found solace in many of the most trying scenes of his future life.' [1] His eldest son Edward was born in the following year, and John Hunter stood godfather.

When writing to his friend, E. Gardner, he speaks of the small house (Chantry Cottage, near the church) which was being put in order for him— of his delight in the countryside, and of the great happiness of his married life. At the same time he writes to the Rev. John Clinch, an old friend, who had been at school with him at Cirencester, a fellow-pupil under John Hunter in London, and who was now in Newfoundland, acting as both clergyman and medical practitioner :

' Berkeley, 7 Feb. 1789.

' My Dearest Friend, . . . I sincerely lament your having been beset by that dreadful fever the typhus, and

---

[1] Baron : *Life of Jenner*, i. 87.

sincerely congratulate you on your recovery. There is
no laying down, I believe, any general mode of treatment
in this disease. A man must be guided by his own
genius ; indeed, without a good portion of this, a
physician must ever cut a poor figure ; and if he should
be a man of fine feelings, he must often be subject to
unpleasant sensations within himself. Something new is
for ever presenting itself. Neither books, lectures, nor
the longest experience are sufficient to store the mind
with the indescribable something a man of our profession
should possess.'

Clinch had apparently offered Jenner's nephew,
George Jenner, some appointment in Newfoundland, for the letter continues :

' George has at length left us to take leave of friends
before he departs for your snowy shores. Your offer was
so liberal that it would have been unjust in me to have
said anything to have damped his ardour for catching
at so good an opportunity of improving his fortune. It
was only in my power to improve his education, and the
progress he made during the time he stayed here was
extremely rapid. You will find him a youth of extraordinary talents. His penetration and discernment are
not limited to his profession . . . as a natural historian
he already ranks high. . . .

' During his absence Henry and myself must fag on as
well as we can . . . Henry is much as you left him : the
same simple, inoffensive lad, and though his mind is
stored with ideas that do him the greatest credit, yet his
general appearance and manner is so very *fifteenish*, that
a poor mortal on the bed of sickness will hardly look up

to him with that eye of confidence and hope that might safely be placed in him.   For it is by appearances, my dear friend, not from a real knowledge of things, that the world forms a judgment.   A look of significance, a peculiar habit, and a very scanty acquaintance with the human machine, will make a man pass current for a great physician.   This you and I know to be an unfortunate fact. . . .

'Pray send me a catalogue of your books, that I may know what medical works may at any time be useful to you . . .

Your ever Faithful and Affectionate friend,
EDWARD JENNER.

'To the Rev. John Clinch,
Newfoundland.'

So Jenner lost the services of his helpful nephew.

Although life at Berkeley was so peaceful, England, during the greater part of Jenner's lifetime, was in the turmoil of war.   Clinch wrote :

'Newfoundland, Dec. 1, 1796.

'You have long ere this received particulars of our late unexpected alarm occasioned by the arrival of Citizen Richery and the powerful squadron under his command . . . in September last ; and as I would not wish to hurt your feelings I shall decline giving you an account of our distressed condition during the time they continued to lord it over us.   I was twice obliged to move my family and part of my effects. . . .

'Just before the French made their appearance on this coast, my friend George and myself had agreed to meet at St. Johns, but our plan was soon disconcerted ; and the whole of my family have been greatly disappointed in the pleasure of his company at Trinity by those unwelcome visitors.'

Another nephew, Stephen Jenner, was lost on the merciless Dorset coast.

As is well known, the Chesil Bank, a steep slope of shingle, extends for many miles in a straight line from Portland with its stone quarries, to Abbotsbury with its great swannery. The sea rolling in from the Atlantic, instead of eating into the coast, has piled up a great wall of shingle a short distance from the land—a protection against its own violence. The pebbles are curiously gradated—as small as marbles at Abbotsbury, some pounds in weight at Portland. Fishermen, forced to land on the Bank at night, know by the size of the stones under their feet on what part of the coast they stand. During a south-west gale the sea beats on the Bank with fury. There is a story of a small ship having been thrown right over it into the still water (the Fleet) yards away on the other side. The sea-swallows nest on it, and the rare wild sea-pea grows on it, out of the reach of hares and rabbits, as it does on a like beach on the Suffolk coast.[1]

---

[1] The fisher folk of Aldeburgh were saved from starvation by this plant when the fishing failed in Queen Mary's reign.

In November 1795, the troopship *Catherine*, one of a fleet on its way to take possession of the French West Indies, after all her canvas had been carried away, was driven on to the Bank. Lieutenant Stephen Jenner, a member of General Abercromby's staff, was on board.

The broken ship was thrown high up on the Bank, and the shingle strewn with battered bodies. Mr. W. F. Shrapnell, an army surgeon stationed at Portland, described the terrible scene. He wrote to Jenner :

'Nov. 22nd, 1795.

' My Dear Friend,—Although exhausted with fatigue I cannot avoid telling you that I have every reason to believe my friend Stephen was unfortunately lost in the *Catherine* transport. I volunteered the command of a party of forty men of our regiment to bury the dead. . . . I have been three days officiating in the melancholy ceremony. I could not distinguish his features . . . but I have lodged in coffins two bodies which I thought resembled him. I will faithfully see them interred, with the bodies of fourteen other officers, with all military honours. . . . The labour I and my party have gone through I look back upon with astonishment. . . . We had every day six miles to walk on a bank of pebbles, one mile an hour, before we could reach the bodies, and then they lay scattered for two miles further. We have buried about two hundred and thirty, but cannot immediately say, as I am much wearied.'

Other ships were lost, and the flagship, with

Sir Ralph Abercromby on board, returned damaged to Spithead.[1]

In 1793 John Hunter—Jenner's tutor, friend, and hero—fell dying while being opposed and contradicted by lesser men in the Board Room of St. George's Hospital ; and so the world lost one whose persevering, philosophical mind, always searching for reasons for the facts he knew, had raised the handicraft of the Barber-surgeons to the science of surgery.

Hunter had long suffered from attacks of *angina pectoris*. Jenner had discovered that in this condition the arteries which supply the muscles of the heart are thickened and inefficient. He received the following letter from Sir Everard Home : [2]

'Leicester Sq., Feb. 1794.

' My dear Sir,—. . . I am well assured that you were sincerely afflicted at the death of your old and most valuable friend, whose death, although we all looked for it, was more sudden than could have been imagined. It is singular that the circumstance you mentioned to me, and were always afraid to touch upon with Mr. Hunter, should have been a particular part of his complaint, as the coronary arteries of the heart were considerably ossified. . . . '

Hunter's great collection—to which Jenner had

---

[1] G. Pinckard : *Notes on the West Indies*, 1806.

[2] Sir Everard Home, F.R.S., whose sister Hunter had married, became a trustee of the Hunterian Collection, wrote many papers in the *Philosophical Transactions*, and destroyed Hunter's MSS.

made many contributions—had been got together chiefly to show the infinite variety of forms, animal and vegetable, in which there had been the mysterious principle of life and growth. It was purchased by the State for £15,000. The Royal College of Surgeons undertook the curatorship, and erected the present magnificent building in Lincoln's Inn Fields.

John Hunter's body was laid to rest in one of the vaults under the church of St. Martin's-in-the-Fields. Sixty-six years later—in January 1859—a notice appeared in *The Times* that all coffins in those vaults would be removed to catacombs under the churchyard, and be inaccessible. Frank Buckland, the well-known naturalist who had been house-surgeon at St. George's Hospital, and—like Jenner—an enthusiastic admirer of Hunter and his works, determined that, if possible, Hunter's body should rest in Westminster Abbey. When vault number 3 was opened some two hundred coffins were to be seen piled up to the ceiling, like books in a packing-case.

Buckland and the vestry surveyor of St. Martin's then spent no fewer than fifteen days in the ' overpowering, sickly effluvia ' of the vaults examining with a bull's-eye lantern each metal plate as the coffins were removed, until, at last, Hunter's name was found. The coffin was put aside, and after many difficulties had been overcome by the College of Surgeons and Buckland, was solemnly reinterred in the Abbey.

Some 3260 coffins were removed from underneath St. Martin's church and then sealed up under the churchyard.[1]

No wonder that in those days women were liable to faint in church.

Anyone who has attended a funeral in Brompton cemetery and has seen a private vault, with its mouldering coffins, must feel that burial in vaults in a crowded city is an anachronism. Buckland was ill for a fortnight after his devoted search, and the vestry surveyor had to leave London for four months.

Towards the end of the year 1793 Jenner had an almost fatal attack of ' typhus ' fever. Whether it was real typhus—the bane of doctors and nurses— or typhoid, which was at that time classed with typhus, it is impossible to say.

He was visited by doctors from Bath and Bristol, but his nephew, George, who was then in England, was his constant and devoted attendant. In a letter to Henry Shrapnell, a neighbour and a friend, Jenner says :

' First fell Henry's wife and sister. . . . It was during my attendance on this case that the venomed arrow

---

[1] Frank Buckland : *Curiosities of Natural History*, series 3, ii. 159.

wounded me. . . . Had it not been for a dreary, weari-
some ride over mountains of ice, no mischief might have
ensued. . . . Great were the efforts of those who kindly
and humanely attended me. Dr. Parry was with me
from Bath five times, Dr. Hicks and Dr. Ludlow as many,
and my friend George was never absent from my bedside.
. . . Henry's infant girl has now the fever ; a servant
maid is dying of it ; and to complete this tragical narra-
tive, five days ago fell poor Henry himself.'

Jenner long felt the effects of his illness.

CHAPTER 3

Jenner as a naturalist. Widespread interest in natural history in Jenner's day. Linnæus. Contemporary naturalists. Hibernation of hedgehogs. Importance of earthworms. The cuckoo ; resemblance of its egg to other eggs in nest. Jenner's observations and experiments. His discovery of the habits of the young cuckoo. Vindication of Jenner's account. His *Migration of Birds*. Morning song of birds.

JENNER was a naturalist,[1] and only by accident the pioneer of vaccination. As a naturalist he was fortunate in being born at a time when, in many countries—especially in England—there was an awakening to an interest in nature.

This was chiefly due to the genius of a Swedish doctor.

In terse language, keeping as far as possible to the classical names, Linnæus had classified the living world—from the highest animal to the simplest flower. Instead of the long descriptive sentence of earlier writers, he had given to each a name consisting of two words : the first the name of the genus, the second the name of the species.

[1] Much of this chapter was written at the request of the Royal College of Physicians, as an introduction to *Jenner's Note Book*, lately published by the College.

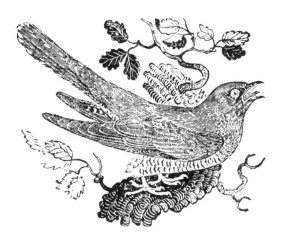

THE CUCKOO.

From a wood-engraving by Jenner's contemporary—
Thomas Bewick of Newcastle.

He had visited England in order to see the Apothecaries' Garden in Chelsea—had walked on Putney Heath—had stayed at Oxford ; so his name and work were well known in this country ; and here during the last half of the eighteenth century—in Jenner's lifetime—the study of natural history took on new life.

During that time *Gleanings in Natural History*, by George Edwards, ' Library Keeper ' to the Royal College of Physicians, was (in 1760) published by the College, in seven quarto volumes. Both the matter and the six hundred coloured plates (chiefly of birds) were so good, that the work was translated into French, German, and Dutch.[1]

On Friday, August 26, 1768, Sir Joseph Banks sailed with Captain Cook on his first and most successful voyage, and brought back many natural history treasures. The British Museum was opened in Bloomsbury in order to house the natural history collection made by a President of the Royal College of Physicians, Sir Hans Sloane. Thomas Pennant, a country squire, wrote a *History of Quadrupeds*, *British Zoology*, *Arctic Zoology*, and much else. ' He's a Whig, sir—a sad dog,' said Dr. Johnson, ' but he observes more things than anyone else.' Daines Barrington, at the same time, wrote on

---

[1] There is a good copy of Edward's work in the College of Physicians library.

natural history. Gilbert White corresponded with both, and compiled his immortal *History of Selborne*. Dr. John Latham of Eltham, like Jenner a pupil of John Hunter's, published in many quarto volumes his *Synopsis of Birds*, with coloured plates etched by himself.

Many collections of butterflies were formed. There was an ' Aurelian Society,' with a collection of butterflies and moths, to which each member contributed—and a Society of London Entomologists. William Jones of Chelsea made beautiful drawings of all the known butterflies of that time, from his own and other collections—no fewer than 1500 figures in all, with descriptions in Latin. The drawings were so accurate that (as Faulkner, in his *History of Chelsea* relates) J. C. Fabricius, the ' Father of Entomology,' named two hundred new species from the drawings alone.[1] In 1925 the bound volumes were given by the present writer to the Oxford Museum.

Long ago the late Professor J. O. Westwood[2]— Hope Professor of Entomology at Oxford—told the writer that quiet, unknown London entomologists of the eighteenth century, chiefly belonging to

---

[1] Thomas Faulkner : *History of Chelsea*, 2nd edition, 1829, i. 84.

[2] Professor J. O. Westwood—a founder, and first Honorary President of the Entomological Society of London—was the author of *British Butterflies and their Transformations*, many other books, and more than three hundred and fifty papers on entomological and archæological subjects.

Huguenot families, were so devoted to their hobby that on Saturday nights in summer they would tramp on foot to such places as Coombe Wood, or even to Darenth Wood in Kent, to pursue their favourite study at daybreak ; and then at nightfall find their way back in time for work—in a different atmosphere—on Monday morning. Perhaps their somewhat puritanical upbringing taught them to prefer the out-of-door interests of the country to the indoor amusements of the City.

Thomas Bewick indulged his love of nature, and of drawing, by publishing his *General History of Quadrupeds*, and, later, his *British Birds*, in two volumes, with his well-known attractive woodcuts— of its own kind the best wood-engraving the world has seen.

John Hunter the surgeon, Curtis the well-known entomologist and botanist, whose *Botanical Magazine* is still published every year, formed, together with others, a Natural History Society ; and a medical student, afterwards Sir James Smith, purchased and brought to England, in twenty-six packing cases, Linnæus' valuable collection of natural history objects, and founded the Linnean Society.

All this took place during the last fifty years of the eighteenth century.

Such a natural history atmosphere no doubt had its influence on Jenner, although there seems to be no record of his having come into contact with, or of his having corresponded with any of those mentioned, except Sir Joseph Banks and John Hunter.

Hunter and Jenner (more than twenty years his junior) continued devoted friends, and the great surgeon, as has been stated, made use of his pupil in obtaining creatures for his menagerie in Brompton, and for his studies in comparative anatomy. The service was willingly rendered.

Jenner carefully preserved letters written by his master—there are many in the library of the College of Surgeons—most of them undated. In these he is requested to procure ' a large porpoise, for love or money '—fossils, salmon-spawn, eels. He is asked : ' What the devil becomes of eels in winter ? ' Hunter wants young blackbirds of different ages, crows' and magpies' nests—with the branches of the tree in which they are built—an old cuckoo, a nest with a cuckoo's egg in it, white hares from Jenner's friends in Newfoundland, bats from the old castle at Berkeley, and more fossils. ' The fossils you sent were none of the best, but I know you did not make them—therefore not your fault.' He is experimenting on the temperature of hibernating animals, and asks Jenner to send him ' more hedgehogs,' ' a colony of them,' for ' one an eagle eat [sic], and a ferret caught the other.' He even wants a bustard, and Jenner sends him one.[1] Hunter writes : ' Dear Jenner, I do not know anyone I would sooner write to than you : I do not know anybody I am so much obliged to.'

Persistent accounts of toads being found embedded and alive in blocks of stone, coal, and wood were recorded both at home and abroad. Hunter tested the truth of the stories. In a letter of his, now in the College of Surgeons, he writes : ' I buried two toads—last August was a twelve month —I opened the grave last October, and they were well and lively. Write me soon.'

Dean Buckland, the geologist, whose collection of fossils enrich both the Oxford and British Museums, made a more scientific experiment. In November 1825, he was Canon of Christ Church, Oxford, living in Tom Quad, where (as Ruskin in *Proeterita*[2] says) Buckland and his family ' gave sap and savour to the whole College.'

---

[1] This great bustard was probably one of the last to be seen on Salisbury Plain. The native race of great bustards lingered on, up till 1838, in the open country in Norfolk and Suffolk. Several appeared in England in 1870, during the Franco-Prussian war, driven over by cold weather and the booming of big guns, and one, a fine male bird, appeared in Norfolk in 1876. Care was taken that it should not be shot, and the late Lord Lilford turned out two female great bustards, hoping that the birds would stay and nest ; but without success. In 1890 another attempt, made by Lord Walsingham and others, to introduce bustards brought from Spain, also failed. The ' open ' country of Norfolk and Suffolk was no longer open enough for bustards. The birds strayed, and were killed in various counties.

[2] J. Ruskin : *Proeterita*, ii. 375.

In November 1825,[1] Buckland placed twelve toads in twelve circular cells excavated in a block of coarse oölitic limestone from Heddington. Glass covers were fitted to the cells, and cemented round the edges with clay.

Twelve other toads were placed in cells cut in hard compact sandstone and covered with glass in the same way. Both blocks were buried three feet deep in the Canon's garden. In a year's time all the toads in the hard sandstone cells were found to be dead, but most of those in the block of porous limestone, which allowed moisture, and, possibly, some air to percolate, were alive.[2]

After receiving Hunter's letter, Jenner made a like experiment, which met with Hunter's approval; but Hunter's executor, Sir Everard Home, although a writer on scientific subjects, lacked the team spirit of the two naturalists, and destroyed Hunter's papers, and with them Jenner's letters.

Fortunately many of the papers had been copied by the Conservator of the College of Surgeons, including numberless records of dissections of creatures—great and small—from elephants to humble bees—one hundred and thirty of mammals alone. Among them is an account of a *whale*!

---

[1] Frank Buckland : *Curiosities of Natural History*, series 1, 46–54.

[2] Some years ago these toads' catacombs were to be seen, together with other stones from the repairs of the Cathedral, in the garden of the house then occupied by the Archdeacon of Oxford. They may still be there.

which Jenner managed to send to Hunter. How it was obtained, or how it travelled to London, is not stated.

Hunter and Jenner jointly investigated the mystery of hibernation among animals. They found that the temperature of hibernating hedgehogs can fall to freezing point—that the heartbeats are lowered to fourteen a minute—that respiration becomes imperceptible—and yet that the blood does not coagulate—that hedgehogs can be thrown about, and subjected to electric shocks, without showing the slightest sign of life, as long as the temperature is kept low.

It is a curious phenomenon—this loss of vitality, unaccompanied by death. It is said to be only the extreme limit of ordinary sleep, so varied, as all know, in depth and length, and so necessary to the renewal of energy. It seems to be a step towards hibernation when small birds, such as wrens and long-tailed tits, which, when awake, require continual feeding to keep up their temperature, sleep, often huddled together for the sake of warmth, for some fourteen hours during the depth of winter—occasionally even in the daytime. The late Lord Lilford writes : ' In very cold weather I have found a family of perhaps a dozen (golden-crested wrens) clustered together for warmth beneath the snow-laden bough of an old yew tree, to the under-surface of which the birds were clinging.'[1] Primitive man, too, must have barricaded himself in his cave, and have slept in darkness for the same time, in winter. Perhaps, if modern man had longer winter sleep he would be the better for it.

Jenner notices a border of 'the night-flowering primrose' with petals 'puckered up and withered,' and so saving their honey during the day, but, after sunset, open, and with 'a considerable number of moths . . . sucking the nutritious fluid prepared for them.'[2] He saw the importance of common earthworms. Sir Humphry Davy wrote :

'. . . I was more disposed to consider the dunghill as useful to the worm, rather than the worm as an agent important to man in the economy of nature : but Dr. Jenner would not allow my reason. He said the earthworms are much under the surface of our meadowlands. . . . They act . . . in furnishing materials for food to the vegetable kingdom, and under the surface, they break the stiff clods in pieces, and . . . divide the soil.'

The patient genius of Darwin elaborated Jenner's observations, and showed the importance of earthworms to vegetation.

---

[1] Lilford : *Birds of Northamptonshire*, i. 135.

[2] The evening primrose was introduced into Europe from America as far back as 1614. By opening its flowers in the evening, and by its strong scent, it attracts the long-tongued moths, on which its fertilisation (by conveyance of pollen) depends.

But Jenner's fame as a naturalist depends on his discovery and careful observation of the extraordinary habits of the young cuckoo.

The male cuckoos, as everyone knows, arrive about the middle of April, and, unless the weather is cold and rainy, utter their well-known call from morning till night. The female cuckoos arrive, in smaller numbers, a few days later, and have a different call. Each female cuckoo, if rivals permit, probably finds her way, as her unknown parents did, to the district in which, as a newly-hatched nestling, she began her most immoral life. She builds no nest—associates with different males—skulks in trees and bushes—marking the nests which small birds around her are building. In about a month's time, she begins, and, if conditions are favourable, continues, every other day, to lay an egg in one of the nests she has chosen.

The cuckoo's egg is small, and, as a rule, has a distinct resemblance to the eggs already in the nest. This must have been long recognised by all birdnesting folk.

Very many years ago—probably it is so now—if a boy at Winchester, during the last weeks of May, or in June, put on his football dress, and waded, up to his waist, among the reed-beds in the river Itchen, he could always find reed-warblers' nests suspended in the reeds, and containing cuckoos' eggs. In colour and markings the cuckoo's egg bore a striking resemblance to the other eggs in the nest.

On the other hand, the cuckoos' eggs, sometimes found in pied-wagtails' nests in a chalk-pit close by, differed, both in colour and markings, from the cuckoos' eggs found in the reed-warblers' nests, but resembled the eggs of the wagtail.

Anyone could see the difference between the two kinds of cuckoos' eggs, but no one could say how the cuckoo managed to colour her eggs, so as to deceive both wagtails and reed-warblers.

Now it has been almost proved that each female cuckoo haunts, more or less, one special kind of victim. One cuckoo victimises reed-warblers, another prefers wagtails, another robins. A cuckoo which had been reared in a wagtail's nest would, for choice, lay her eggs in a wagtail's nest.

On arriving in the country (probably the county and district) of her birth, the cuckoo, as she skims over the fields, would recognise the look and the anxious notes of the birds which she would remember as her foster-parents. She might even see the very pair of wagtails which, during some previous summer, were occupied, all the day long, in bringing food to her capacious mouth. Naturally, she would choose the nests of birds of that kind.

Another cuckoo, brought up by reed-warblers, would recognise the incessant song of the reed-warblers by the river-side, and choose their nests. Thus, like other rogues, cuckoos probably specialise in the dupes they select, and the choice remains hereditary.

So, through countless ages, those cuckoos' eggs which had some resemblance to the eggs already in the nest have been accepted by the victim, while those which had no resemblance have been liable to rejection; and the copying of the victim's eggs has, no doubt, improved with time.

In England there is one marked exception to this rule. A cuckoo's egg found in a hedge-sparrow's nest bears no resemblance whatever to the greeny-blue eggs of the host. The meek, little, plainly dressed hedge-sparrow, hopping on the gravel path, and, at the sound of a footstep, retreating like a mouse to its hedge, accepts without question the strange egg, so unlike its own, and becomes a favourite dupe of the cuckoo. Jenner records in his *Note Book* that even a large blackbird's egg, which he had put in a hedge-sparrow's nest, was hatched, and that the young blackbird was brought up by the hedge-sparrows.

In Finland, however, those cuckoos which choose redstarts' and whinchats' nests, have been compelled by centuries of ' selection ' to produce eggs which match the blue eggs of their victims—as can be seen in the collection of cuckoos' eggs in the Natural History Museum in Kensington.

In the North of England, where the titlark, which builds its nest on the ground, is a favourite victim, the cuckoo has been seen to lay her egg directly into the nest of that bird, and carry off one of the eggs already there. She has been photographed in the act. When a less accessible nest is chosen, the egg must of necessity be laid outside, and be introduced into the nest by the bill. It is all done deftly and quickly—the work of an accomplished pickpocket.

The eggs are hatched, and the young cuckoo alone survives. How it managed to get rid of its companions was not known until Jenner's discovery was published.

John Hunter had asked Jenner to send him a ' true and particular account of the cuckoo, and as far as possible under your own eye ' ; [1] so Jenner, with the help of his nephew Henry, made careful observations of nests on a farm belonging to his aunt, where he had spent some time as a boy. This often involved a walk of four or five miles. Many nests containing a cuckoo's egg were watched, and experiments were made. These are recorded in *Jenner's Note Book*. It

[1] Baron : *Life of Edward Jenner*, i. 69.

resulted in a paper,[1] which John Hunter handed to the Royal Society in July 1787, describing the murderous activity of the newly-hatched cuckoo.

It is a long paper. Jenner records not one, but many observations and experiments. He says that the song of the male bird is well known—that the note of the female is ' like the cry of a dabchick '— that the female is often attended by many males ; that she does not begin to lay until after the middle of May—that the hedge-sparrow's nest is the one generally chosen in his district.

In a hedge-sparrow's nest, which he examined in June 1787, he says that to his ' astonishment ' he saw the young cuckoo, though ' so lately hatched,' in the act of turning out its companion.

' The mode of accomplishing this was very curious. The little animal with the assistance of its rump and wings, contrived to get the bird ' (the young hedge-sparrow) ' upon its back, and making a lodgement for the burden by elevating its elbows, clambered backward with it up the side of the nest till it reached the top, where, resting for a moment, it threw off its load with a jerk, and quite disengaged it from the nest. It remained in this situation a short time feeling about with the

---

[1] *Philosophical Transactions*, 1788, pp. 219-237. It was written in a cottage belonging to Mr. Hicks at Eastington. The observations on the cuckoo were chiefly made at a farm belonging to Jenner's aunt, Mrs. Hooper, at Clapton, near Berkeley.

extremities of its wings, as if to be convinced whether the business was properly executed, and then dropped into the nest again.

' With the extremities of its wings, I have often seen it examine, as it were, an egg and nestling before it began its operations ; and the nice sensibility which these parts appeared to possess, seemed sufficiently to compensate the want of sight which as yet it was destitute of. I afterwards put in an egg, and this, by a similar process, was conveyed to the edge of the nest, and thrown out.

' These experiments I have since repeated several times in different nests, and have always found the young cuckoo disposed to act in the same manner. . . . It is wonderful to see the extraordinary exertions of the young cuckoo, when it is two or three days old, if a bird be put into the nest too weighty for it to lift out. In this state it seems ever restless and uneasy ; but this disposition for turning out its companions begins to decline from the time it is two or three till it is about twelve days old, when, as far as I have hitherto seen, it ceases. Indeed, the disposition for throwing out the eggs appears to cease a few days sooner ; for I have frequently seen the young cuckoo, after it had been hatched nine or ten days, remove a nestling that had been placed in the nest with it, when it suffered an egg put there at the same time to remain unmolested.

' The singularity of its shape is well adapted to these purposes : for, different from other newly-hatched birds, its back from the *scapulæ* downwards is very broad, with a considerable depression in the middle. This depression seems formed by nature for giving a more secure lodgement to the egg of the hedge-sparrow, or its young one, when the young cuckoo is moving either of them from the nest. When it is about twelve days old this cavity is quite filled up, and then the back assumes the shape of nestling birds in general.'

It is a wonderful story—this slow evolution through the ages of all that helped the parasitic life of the cuckoo, the rapidly growing ability of its two-days-old offspring to throw the young hedge-sparrow out of its nest, and the fashioning of a temporary depression on the murderous infant's back—an egg-cup for the unhatched hedge-sparrow's egg, or freshly-hatched bird, about to be jettisoned !

Jenner's paper was sent to the Royal Society. What a shaking of heads there must have been when the council received it ! Although Sir Joseph Banks, the President, who knew Jenner, may have believed his statements, it was agreed that, as further observations were being made, the acceptance of the paper should be deferred. Banks then wrote the following courteous and diplomatic letter to Jenner :

'Soho Square, July 7, 1787.

'Sir,—. . . In consequence of your having discovered that the young cuckoo, and not the parent bird, removes the eggs and young from the nest in which it is deposited, the council thought it best to give you a full scope for altering it as you shall choose. Another year we shall be glad to receive it again, and print it. . . . Mr. Hunter has given us a most excellent paper on the genus of whales.

I am, Sir,
Your most obedient and
very humble servant,
JOSEPH BANKS.'

Banks, it may be noted, in his official capacity, uses to the full the artificial and untruthful ending to his letter which was in use at that time. There is an interesting note on this style of writing in Smyth's *Lives of the Berkeleys.* Its mock humility apparently came from France. Smyth says:

'At this time (about 1575) the anticke and apish gestures since used in salutations, nor the French garbes of cringinge were not yet arrived. The subscription of letters "your humble servant" hath, since that time, almost driven "your loving friend" quite out of England.'

It is curious that, in a truthful nation, the custom should have lasted so long. Perhaps there is a slight stand-offishness in the English character which at times finds the formality of the 'subscription' useful.

Jenner's paper was read before the Royal Society the following year.

In a letter to the Rev. Dr. Worthington, Jenner writes : ' I am sure the cuckoo has nothing to do with hatching, as the adults are off while a great number of eggs remain unhatched.' The old cuckoos are off in June and July, leaving their insatiable young to be brought up by small, devoted foster-mothers, and then to find their own way south as soon as their wings are strong enough to carry them.[1]

It is difficult to imagine the method by which an infant cuckoo hatched in a robin's or redstart's nest in a hole in a wall, and at a distance of some inches from the entrance, manages to get rid of its foster-brothers—when hoisted to the brim of the nest they would not fall out. Further observations by out-of-door naturalists, like Jenner, are wanted.

Jenner, in his *Note Book*, mentions the large number of eggs which he finds in the bodies of female cuckoos. He was probably the first to notice this. In the great Hunterian Museum in Lincoln's Inn Fields there is a most carefully prepared dissection of a cuckoo by Jenner, showing one fully developed egg and a large number of smaller eggs of varying size.

It has lately been proved that a cuckoo is capable of laying more than twenty eggs in one season. Fortunately there must be great mortality

[1] A short time ago a young cuckoo, in Buckinghamshire, was labelled with an aluminium ring. Eighteen months afterwards its body was brought to a missionary in the French Cameroons by a native, who, on shooting it with his bow and arrow, found that it was wearing a magic ring. So Buckinghamshire cuckoos winter in the Cameroons.

among the eggs and young of this destructive bird. If one-fourth of the eggs laid by cuckoos made old birds, many more young robins, hedge-sparrows, wagtails, titlarks, and other small birds would be ruthlessly thrown overboard, and some species possibly exterminated.

Probably the reason why the harmless little hedge-sparrow, beloved by gardeners and all country folk—no relation of the coarser, commoner house-sparrow—content to feed on such minute insects as it finds in a garden rubbish-heap—is not more abundant, is that it accepts without criticism any kind of cuckoo's egg, and devotes the best days of the summer to feeding the voracious murderer. Many thousands of young hedge-sparrows must be thus slaughtered every year, and the parents prevented from rearing a second brood.

On a country walk, many must have noticed the extraordinary resemblance an old cuckoo bears to a sparrow-hawk, and the young cuckoo to a kestrel. It is as true an instance of what naturalists call ' mimicry ' as is the copying of a butterfly, distasteful to birds and lizards, by another, but edible, species of butterfly ; or the copying of hornets and wasps by ' clear-wing ' moths. What is the advantage to the bird of this disguise ?

It has been suggested that the hawk-like appearance and manner of the cuckoo is useful in driving a sitting victim from its eggs, and that other hawks would not attack a bird that looked like one of themselves ; but it seems to the writer that the chief advantage of the hawk-like appearance is that it helps the cuckoo to find nests.

During the fresh, pleasant early hours of a June day, when disturbing man is still asleep, and all nature is free to enjoy the ' top of the morning ' and its sweet air, the hawk-like cuckoo, gliding over hedge, and heath, and garden wall, excites violent protests from each nest-building bird. The birds thus betray their nests, and enable the cuckoo to note, not only the whereabouts and condition of nests, and prospect of eggs, but the nature of the owners. A cuckoo must know the state of suitable nests which are being built in her district long before she makes use of them ; and the agitated owners involuntarily help her in the search.

The year after Jenner's paper appeared, Gilbert White published his *Natural History of Selborne.* He had been wondering how many eggs a cuckoo was capable of laying. In a letter [1] written in 1770 he says :

' I think the matter might easily be determined whether a cuckoo lays one, or two, or more eggs in a season by opening a female during the laying time. I will endeavour to get a hen to examine.'

[1] *History of Selborne.* Letter 5 to Daines Barrington.

E

But the elusive hen-cuckoos seem to have escaped Gilbert White's gun, for the subject is not mentioned again. In the meantime, Jenner had shown that the bird was capable of laying a large number of eggs.

The cuckoo has been described as a useful bird, because, always hungry, it will eat hairy caterpillars, which no other bird will touch. Its large stomach has been found with a fur lining composed of caterpillars' hair. But, as many must have noticed, hairy caterpillars appear in gardens chiefly in the late summer, at a time when most of the cuckoos have gone, so the good cuckoos do must be infinitesimal.

Descriptions of the cuckoo feeding *chiefly* on *hairy* caterpillars must be exaggerated. Jenner, in his *Note Book*, gives the contents of the stomachs of four cuckoos. One stomach contained three *hairy* caterpillars—another 'caterpillars, small beetles, and other insects'—the third and fourth *many* ' *smooth* ' caterpillars, beetles, flies, and other insects—the food of numberless other birds.[1]

Cuckoos have been kept in aviaries, and even when tame remain ill-conditioned and unsociable. The late Lord Lilford found them ' sulky, greedy, spiteful.' [2]

As was to be expected, Jenner's extraordinary

---

[1] *Jenner's Note Book*, pp. 21, 22, 23.
[2] Lilford : *Coloured Figures of British Birds*, ii. 22.

story has been discredited by many. Waterton [1] states the case for the sceptics. In his essay on *The Jay*, he writes that an American friend had asked him his opinion on the ' English account concerning the young cuckoo.' Waterton answered :

' No bird in the creation could perform such an astonishing feat under such embarrassing circumstances. The young cuckoo cannot, by any means, support its own weight during the first day of its existence. Of course, then, it is utterly incapable of clambering, rump foremost, up the steep side of a hedge-sparrow's nest, with the additional weight of a young hedge-sparrow on its back. Add to this, that an old bird, the young of which are born blind, always remains on the nest during the whole of the day on which the chick is excluded from the shell. . . . The account carries its own condemnation, no matter by whom related, or by whom received. I would much rather believe the story of baby Hercules throttling snakes.'

And again, in a letter to G. Ord, he writes, ' You are quite right with regard to Jenner's preposterous account of the young cuckoo. He never saw what he relates.' [2]

But the late Professor Alfred Newton, of Cambridge, in his ' Dictionary of Birds,' [3] says truly :

' A wholly unjustifiable attempt has lately been made to impugn Jenner's accuracy. His observations as printed

---

[1] Charles Waterton's *Essays*. Edited by Sir Norman Moore, M.D., F.R.C.P., 1871, p. 317.
[2] Charles Waterton's *Essays*, p. 555.   [3] *Dictionary of Birds*, i. 120.

in the "Philosophical Transactions" for 1788 have been corroborated by others in the most minute detail.'

Photography, too, has confirmed Jenner's observations. An interesting series of photographs of the young cuckoo's method of eviction was shown [1] at the Linnean Society by Mr. F. H. Lancum. A young cuckoo—thirty-six hours old—was to be seen tilting with its wing a yellow-hammer's egg on to its hollowed back—grasping with its large feet the perpendicular side of the nest, hoisting the egg, almost as heavy as itself, up to the edge of the nest, and then, with a vigorous effort, throwing it out. The operation, which occupied less than a minute, was continually repeated when the egg was replaced. It was all exactly the process which Jenner had described a century and a half earlier.

Lately, a careful preparation of the skeleton of a young cuckoo, showing the structures involved in the temporary distortion of its back in order to keep the egg in position for ejectment, has been placed in the Museum of the College of Surgeons by the curator, R. H. Burne, F.R.S.

Soon after Hunter's death, natural history studies were put aside, and Jenner devoted himself entirely to his campaign in the cause of vaccination. Towards the end of life he turned to his old love,

[1] On December 19, 1920.

and tried to finish a paper he had been asked to write for the Royal Society, on the *Migration of Birds*. At that time Sir Humphry Davy [1] was President, having succeeded Sir Joseph Banks, who had held that office with distinction for forty-one years. On Jenner's death, Davy, who had accompanied Jenner on some of his natural history investigations, found, and presented to the Royal Society, the unfinished paper. [2]

In reading it we must remember that in Jenner's time it was believed that some of the birds which disappeared in autumn could not possibly cross the sea, but that they hibernated, as bats do, in cracks, crevices, and holes in rocks and buildings, throughout the winter months ; that the land-rail, for instance—a bird with wingless relations—which apparently finds some difficulty in flying more than a few yards at a time, could not possibly cross the channel.

Gilbert White, although he had seen flocks of swallows flying out towards the sea in autumn, believed that some of them hibernated. He wrote (Feb. 28, 1769) :

'Swallows seem to lay themselves up, and to come forth on a warm day, as bats do continually, of a warm

---

[1] It should never be forgotten that Davy took out no patent for the miner's safety lamp which bears his name, but allowed it to be freely copied at home and abroad.

[2] *Philosophical Transactions*, 1824.

evening, after they have disappeared for weeks . . . We are yet not quite certain to what regions they migrate ; and . . . some do not migrate at all.'

He continually expresses that opinion.

Dr. Beddoes, a well-known lecturer on chemistry at Oxford, actually believed the old legend that swallows, during winter, hid in the mud of the lakes and ponds which they haunted in the summer. Even Gilbert White [1] seems to have thought this possible ; for he writes of house-martins hatched in the autumn :

' Did these small, weak birds shift their quarters at this late season of the year . . . ? Is it not more probable that the next church, ruin, chalk-cliff . . . *lake, or pool* may *become their hybernaculum* ? '

Jenner, in his paper, points out that many know, from their own observation, that birds can take long flights—that his nephew, Lieutenant Jenner, on his way to Newfoundland, saw a hobby-hawk and a swallow, when more than a hundred leagues out at sea—that another nephew (the Rev. G. C. Jenner), when crossing the Atlantic, saw an owl ' gliding over the ocean with as much apparent ease as if it had been seeking for a mouse in its native fields,' [2] that wild geese have been ' fre-

---

[1] Gilbert White : *History of Selborne.* Letter 38 to Thomas Pennant.

[2] Endless observations of nature could then be made from sailing ships ; few are now possible from the top deck of a great steamship.

quently shot in Newfoundland with their crops full of maize,' which must have been eaten far away—that pigeons ' near the Hague, make daily marauding excursions to Norfolk ' to feed on vetches—that if birds hibernated, they would appear in the spring—as hibernating animals do—' in a languid state—their fat all absorbed,' but they arrive in good condition.

In answer to Dr. Beddoes, Jenner mentions that even diving birds are drowned if they become entangled in fishing-nets, or come up under ice in winter.

He throws light on the problem of the land-rail :

' The apparent incapacity of the land-rail to perform the task of migration has often been . . . strongly adduced as a presumptive argument in favour of the hibernating system. . . . It must be admitted that a superficial examination of the habits of this bird tends to favour its incapacity for so great an exploit, as it often rises from the ground like an animated lump, and seems with difficulty to take a flight of a hundred yards. . . . Should it be forced upon the wing by the pursuit of a hawk, the velocity of its flight, and the rapidity of its evolutions to avoid the enemy, will at once appear. . . . *This is no very rare exhibition.*   Necessity here, as in migration, becomes the parent of exertion.'

How few of those now living in our urbanised island have had the rare chance of watching a peregrine in pursuit of a corn-crake ! Jenner's observation is, no doubt, correct. The late Lord Lilford, in his excellent account of the birds of Northamptonshire,[1] writes :

' No one who has only seen these birds (land-rails) flushed from thick covert, with legs hanging, and apparently laboured flight for perhaps a hundred yards, would believe in their power of rapid, sustained, and lofty progress through the air ; but it has happened to us on one occasion to see a land-rail passing high overhead, apparently travelling for pleasure ; and again, we remember one of these birds that, having been flushed twice, fairly took the air, and went quite out of our sight at a great height, and with a speed equal to that of the ordinary flight of a Wild Duck.'

In Yarrell's well-known *History of British Birds* [2] it is related that a land-rail rested on a ship two hundred miles out in the Atlantic.

Jenner shows that birds by their extraordinary sense of direction, return to the spot where they nested the previous year. He removed two claws from the feet of each of the swifts nesting in the roof of a farm-house. Next year he examined them when at roost, and found the marked birds nesting there. They returned the next year, and the year after.

He believed the impulse for nesting in a place

[1] Lilford : *Birds of Northamptonshire*, 1895, i. 318.
[2] Yarrell's *History of British Birds*, revised by Howard Saunders, edition 4, iii. 139.

advantageous for their offspring to be the chief cause of migration in the spring. That done, the migrants are ready to leave. Each pair of swifts has reared its two young ones by August. Then, although the weather may be warm and food abundant, they go.

In his unfinished paper he writes of the order in which birds begin their morning songs. Early morning wakefulness does not trouble the old naturalist :

'First the robin, not the lark, as has been imagined, at twilight, begins his lonely song. How sweetly does this harmonise with the sweet dawning of day ! . . . then up starts the lark : and with him a variety of sprightly songsters whose notes are in perfect correspondence with the gaiety of the morning. The general warbling continues with, now and then, an interruption by the transient croak of the raven, or the screaming of the swift . . . The nightingale unwearied . . . joins in the general harmony. The thrush, placed on the summit of some lofty trees . . . utters its loud notes . . . softened by distance before they reach the ears. The mellow blackbird seeks the inferior branches . . . Thus we see that birds have no inconsiderable share in harmonising some of the most beautiful and interesting scenes in nature.'

So the birds sang Jenner's requiem.

CHAPTER 4

THROUGHOUT the world, in Jenner's day, smallpox was a dreaded and loathsome disease. It was not only dangerous to life, but it left its survivors with scarred faces—sometimes blind, deaf, or insane.

Inoculation (long practised in the East, and to a slight extent in Wales and Scotland) had been introduced by its enthusiastic promoter, Lady Mary Wortley Montagu. It was not a success. Inoculated smallpox was not always a mild disease ; it was occasionally fatal, and it kept smallpox alive

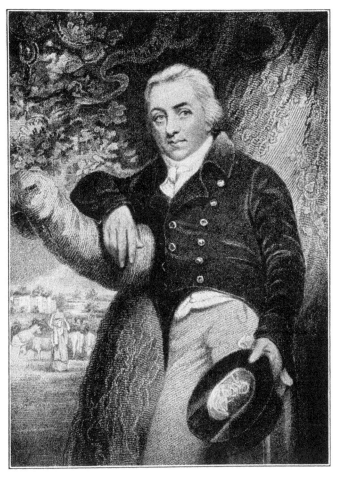

EDWARD JENNER, M.D., F.R.S.

From an engraving by R. Page.

in the country. Those who had not been inoculated were continually exposed to the infection.

So in Jenner's time, when inoculation was generally practised, mortality from smallpox had increased. In 1752 there were no fewer than 3538 deaths from smallpox in England ; and in Paris the mortality was even higher. In France the practice of inoculation became illegal in 1762, but in England it was allowed to continue until 1840.[1]

In Russia the Empress Catherine invited Dr. (afterwards Baron) Dimsdale to St. Petersburg to inoculate herself and her son. The practice spread, and with it the infection. One child in every seven died of smallpox throughout Russia.[2]

Jenner, like others of his time, endured the full ritual considered necessary for inoculation. Fosbroke,[3] who knew him well, writes :

' He was a fine ruddy boy, and, at eight years of age, was, with many others, put under a preparatory process for inoculation with the smallpox. This preparation lasted six weeks. He was bled to ascertain whether his blood was fine ; was purged repeatedly, till he became emaciated and feeble ; was kept on a very low diet . . . and dosed with a diet-drink to sweeten the blood. After this barbarism of human veterinary practice, he was removed to one of the usual inoculation stables, and haltered up with others, in a terrible state of disease.'

[1] Baron : *Life of Edward Jenner*, i. 231.
[2] J. Moore : *History of Smallpox*, p. 286—a book dedicated to Jenner.
[3] F. J. Fosbroke : *Berkeley Manuscripts*, p. 221.

He was a sensitive child, and the effect of all this preparation and inoculation was that for a long time he was unable to enjoy sound sleep, and was haunted by imaginary noises.

So when, a few years later, as a medical student at Sodbury, Jenner heard a young country-woman say, ' I cannot take smallpox, for I have had cowpox,' the remark was never forgotten. He mentioned it to John Hunter, who spoke of the tradition in his lectures. He alluded to the subject at the local medical societies ; but the evidence was considered ' inconclusive and unsatisfactory.' His hearers became tired of the subject. They must have known that milkmaids were celebrated for their clear complexions and unscarred faces, but their knowledge carried them no further.

Jenner continued his investigations. He was in an ideal part of the country for such inquiries. The Vale of Berkeley was celebrated for its dairies. Jenner himself had a small farm—became a member of the Board of Agriculture,[1] and was friendly with all the agricultural community.

He showed Sir Everard Home, and Mr. Cline, Surgeon to St. Thomas's Hospital, a drawing of the ' cow-pox' vesicle, and spoke to others about it; but it was not until 1796 that he had an opportunity of proving that it was possible to vaccinate a human being with lymph taken from another person's arm.

[1] Baron : *Life of Edward Jenner*, ii. 407.

In that year a milkmaid, Sarah Nelmes, was found to have a hand which had been infected while milking a cow. A drawing was made of it—probably by Jenner's nephew, Stephen, who was a good artist—and then a healthy boy, James Phipps, was vaccinated in two places with lymph taken from one of the vesicles on the girl's hand. Later on, the boy was tested by inoculation, and proved to be invulnerable to smallpox. The occasion was historic. The 14th of May—the day of the vaccination—became, and continued for many years, the date of an annual festival in Berlin.

For Jenner it was a serious moment, when a vision of the magnitude of his discovery—the means of rescuing generations yet unborn from a miserable fate—appeared to him—compelling him—a man now well past middle age, to give up a life of comparative ease, and become, for the remainder of his days, a missionary of vaccination.

He wrote :

' The joy I felt at the prospect before me of being the instrument destined to take away from the world one of its greatest calamities . . . was so excessive that I sometimes found myself in a kind of reverie.'

For a time Jenner was hindered in his experiments by the disappearance of cow-pox from the dairies. It then reappeared, and vaccination was carried out by him with all the genius for taking pains, and accurate observation, which he had shown in watching the habits of young cuckoos.

He was advised not to send a record of his observations to the Royal Society, which was prepared to refuse it, but to publish it as a pamphlet; and as a pamphlet it appeared in 1798 : *An Inquiry into the Causes and Effects of Variolæ Vacciniæ. A disease discovered in some of the Western Counties of England*—some seventy pages, with excellent illustrations. In it he states his belief that the disease called ' grease ' in horses, swine-pox, and cow-pox are identical, and that they are modified forms of smallpox. He gives several instances in which those infected with cow-pox, either intentionally or unintentionally, became immune from inoculated smallpox.

In 1798 Jenner stayed in London for three months, hoping to find someone on whom he could demonstrate the beneficial effects of vaccination, but no patient was forthcoming. Smallpox inoculation—often by unskilful hands—was being carried on everywhere, occasionally with fatal results, but no one could be found who would submit to vaccination.

Fortunately, Jenner had left with Mr. Cline some lymph, which had been taken from the arm of a child. With this lymph, dried, and kept in a quill for three months, a boy in St. Thomas's Hospital, suffering from hip disease, was vaccinated on the hip. The vaccination might fail, but the counter-irritation might be useful. The child, when inoculated, proved to be immune from smallpox.

Mr. Cline and Sir W. Farquhar (Physician-in-Ordinary to the Prince of Wales) now tried in vain to persuade Jenner to take a house in Grosvenor Square, promising him £10,000 a year. But the brilliant prospect failed to attract him. He still clung to the ideals of peace and simplicity which had recalled him to Berkeley in his youth. In a touching letter he writes to a friend : [1]

' It is very clear from your representation that there is now an opening in town for any physician whose reputation stood fair in the public eye. But here, my dear friend, is the rub. Shall I, who, even in the morning of my days, sought the lowly and sequestered paths of life —the valley, and not the mountain ; shall I, now my evening is fast approaching, hold myself up as an object for fortune and for fame ? What stock should I add to my little fund of happiness ?

' My fortune, with what flows in from my profession, is sufficient to gratify my wishes ; indeed, so limited is my ambition, and that of my nearest connections, that were I precluded from further practice I should be enabled to obtain all I want.

' And as for fame, what is it ? A gilded butt, for ever pierced with the arrows of malignancy. The name of John Hunter stamps this observation with the signature of truth. . . .

' On the one hand, unwilling to come to town myself

[1] Baron : *Life of Edward Jenner*, i. 155.

for the sake of practice, and on the other fearful that the practice (of vaccination) I have recommended may fall into the hands of those who are incapable of conducting it, I am thrown into a state that was at first not perceptible as likely to happen to me ; for, indeed, I am not callous to all the feelings of those wounds which, from misrepresentation, might fall on my reputation . . .

'How few are capable of conducting physiological experiments ! I am fearful that before we thoroughly understand what is cow-pox matter, and what is not, some confusion may arise ; for which I shall, unjustly, be made answerable . . .'

So Jenner was torn in two by conflicting emotions. He had no wish to live in London, but at the same time he foresaw the harm that might be done to the cause of vaccination by unskilful and unscrupulous vaccinators, and he longed to be on the spot where he could best teach its principles and practice.

His wife's health was at this time causing him some anxiety, so he went to Cheltenham, and spent the next few months between that town and Berkeley, collecting further information on vaccination. Requests were continually being received for lymph, but in the meantime cow-pox seemed to have disappeared from Gloucestershire dairies, and lymph was unobtainable. There were fewer inoculated dairymen to infect the cows.

Vaccination then met with a check. Dr. Woodville had been distributing lymph from the smallpox hospital. It was sent all over Europe as Jenner's lymph, but it produced a general, mild smallpox eruption. Jenner explained that it had been contaminated with smallpox virus, and so fell out with Woodville. Harm, too, was being done by lymph taken from vaccine vesicles in their later septic stage.

Nevertheless vaccination slowly made its way. A Mr. Fermor, finding that milkers in Oxfordshire were protected from smallpox, invited George Jenner to bring lymph, and vaccinate 326 persons in the neighbourhood. Of these 173 were afterwards inoculated with smallpox as a test, and proved immune.

Early in 1800 Jenner returned to London, and stayed in Adam Street, Adelphi, his chief object being to inquire about the management of an institution for gratuitous vaccination which had been started by Dr. Woodville, Dr. Pearson, and others, and for which royal patronage had been obtained. Jenner had not been consulted in the matter, but he was asked if he would give his name as an ' Extra Consulting Physician.' This he could not do, for he disapproved of the practice carried on at the Institution.

Baron [1] says :

' The conduct of the individuals who framed the Institution proved that the cause of vaccination could not be safely committed to their hands ; and that an

---

[1] Baron : *Life of Edward Jenner*, i. 370.

establishment which had been organised as this was, could not receive his sanction without his appearing to abandon those truths which he had advanced respecting the nature of vaccination.'

The Duke of York and the Earl of Egremont, who had been patrons of this Institution, afterwards withdrew from it.

That year Jenner was presented to the King by Lord Berkeley—and also to the Queen and to the Prince of Wales, all of whom were interested in the question of vaccination.

It had become a popular subject for conversation. Charles James Fox asks Jenner what the vaccination vesicle is like, and Jenner describes it as a pearl on a pink rose petal. Jane Austen in a letter to her sister (November 20, 1800) writes [1] that after a dinner-party ' there was a whist and a casino table, and six outsiders. Mat Robinson fell asleep, and James and Augusta alternately read Dr. Jenner's pamphlet on the cow-pox.' [2]

A letter, written at that time by a doctor at Hadleigh, in Suffolk, to Jenner, shows that the practice was extending in the Eastern Counties. It ran :

' I am happy to inform you that in spite of ignorant prejudice, and wilful misrepresentation, this wonderful

---

[1] Jane Austen's *Letters*, 1932, i. 93.
[2] A new edition had just been published, and also a small pamphlet of instructions for vaccination.

discovery is spreading far and wide in this county. The first people we vaccinated in Hadleigh were pelted, and drove into their houses, if they appeared out.

' We have now persuaded our apothecary to vaccinate the whole town (700 or 800 persons).'

Jenner spent the early part of 1800 in London, promoting the cause of vaccination (as opposed to inoculation), attending conferences, medical societies, and public meetings.

He writes to his friend Mr. H. Shrapnell :

' I have not made half my calls yet in town, although I fag from eleven till four. . . . The death of three children under inoculation with the smallpox will probably give that practice the Brutus-stab here, and sink for ever the tyrant smallpox.'

In June, with his nephew George, he left London for Berkeley. At Oxford, on the way, he was introduced to the Vice-Chancellor, and gladly received the following testimonial, signed by Sir C. Pegge, Reader in Anatomy, Mr. Grosvenor, Surgeon to the Radcliffe Infirmary, Dr. Williams, Professor of Botany, and Dr. Wall, Professor of Chemistry :

' We . . . are fully satisfied, upon the conviction of our own observation, that the cow-pox is not only an infinitely milder disease than the smallpox, but has the advantage of *not being contagious,* and is an effectual remedy against the smallpox.'

Jenner's pamphlet had now reached America. It met with much the same reception as had been given it elsewhere. A few, including the able and cultivated President, John Adams, saw the truth and importance of his statements—some expressed no opinion—the greater number treated the whole subject with ridicule. Dr. Waterhouse, Professor of Medicine at Cambridge, Massachusetts, after many attempts, procured lymph from Dr. Haygarth of Bath, and vaccinated his children, who became immune from inoculated smallpox.

Then the tide turned. There was a wild rush for vaccination throughout America—Jenner's precautions were neglected, and shirt-sleeves, stiffened with discharge from ' bad arms,' were sold in strips and used by both medicos and quacks with unhappy results. Later, Dr. Waterhouse received clean lymph from Jenner. President Jefferson, his family, relations, and neighbours were all successfully vaccinated, and credit was restored.

War and revolution had delayed vaccination in Paris, but this year (1800) a translation of Jenner's pamphlet into French went through three editions in seven months.

At the same time the Medical Society of Plymouth, where Mr. Dunning was a warm advocate of vaccination, requested Jenner to sit for his portrait to Northcote. Baron considered it a good likeness. A print made from a mezzotint of the painting forms the frontispiece of this book.

The following year a mission, under Drs. Marshall and Walker, was sent by the British Government to vaccinate the fleet and garrisons at Gibraltar and Malta. At Minorca smallpox was ' proceeding with rapidity, patients daily falling victims to its horrid ravages.' The plague was stopped and blessings were ' called down on the head of Jenner.' At Malta, lately captured by Nelson from the French, several seamen on the *Alexander* and other ships had died of smallpox ; so a Jennerian Institute was established at Malta to which the inhabitants thankfully resorted for vaccination.

At Palermo, in Sicily, where eight thousand persons had died of smallpox during the preceding year, vaccination was welcomed. Processions of men, women, and children for vaccination were conducted through the streets, headed by a priest.

As a token of their admiration for his work, a gold medal was presented to Jenner from the medical officers of the Mediterranean Fleet.

Dr. Marshall stayed three months at Malta. In the words of the Governor, ' he rendered the most essential service to the inhabitants by the introduction of vaccine inoculation, by which the ravages of the smallpox so dreadful in this climate, were prevented.'

In 1801 that brave general, Sir Ralph Abercromby, always careful of the health of his men, was ordered to Egypt to oust the army left there by Napoleon as a step towards India. Dr. Walker accompanied the expedition, vaccinated all the soldiers and seamen, and thus contributed materially to the success of the campaign.

From Paris the practice of vaccination soon spread to Spain. The Royal Economical Society of Madrid elected Jenner an honorary member. Lord Holland,[1] who was then in Spain, forwarded their diploma through his secretary, Mr. Allen, who wrote :

' There is no country likely to receive more benefit from your labours than Spain ; for on the one hand the mortality among children from smallpox, and its consequences, has always been very great ; and on the other hand the inoculation for the cow-pox has been received with the same enthusiasm here as in the rest of Europe : though I am sorry to add that the inoculation of the spurious sort has proved fatal to many children at Seville, who have fallen victims to the smallpox after they had been pronounced secure from that disease . . . as one of the many proofs of the estimation in which the cow-pox and its discoverer are held in Spain, I have enclosed a small engraving . . . to be prefixed to a dissertation . . . to be published by the Royal Society of Medicine (of Madrid).'

In spite of the serious failure of some of the Spanish lymph, Spain was so convinced of the

[1] 3rd Lord Holland (of Macaulay's *Essays*).

efficacy of vaccination that in 1803, under the King of Spain's orders, a philanthropic naval expedition was fitted out, in order to diffuse vaccination throughout the Spanish possessions in both the Old and New Worlds.

The expedition sailed from Cadiz with twenty-two unvaccinated children on board, in order to keep up the strain of lymph. From the Canary Islands it sailed to Porto Rico, where it divided into two branches—one for South America—one for Havana and Yucatan. It was away three years ; Buenos Ayres, Mexico, Peru, Teneriffe, Philippine Islands, and other Spanish colonies were visited. Members of the expedition were everywhere received with enthusiasm—even by the Indian tribes, who had been decimated by smallpox, which they looked upon as the most terrible affliction heaven could send them. Infected persons were banished to hovels, unattended and with little food. Whole families were wiped out. In three different places indigenous cow-pox was discovered among the cattle, and twenty-six more children were taken on board to keep up the supply of lymph.

It was then decided to sail to Canton, and to teach the Chinese to vaccinate. 'In China,' wrote Sir J. Barrow, 'smallpox has usually been attended with the most fatal effects.' So the

expedition was welcomed, and a treatise on vaccination was printed in Chinese, and that by a people
strenuously opposed to every innovation.

' Jennerian ' lymph reached India by a circuitous
route. Jenner was anxious that it should be sent
to India, and to Ceylon, where smallpox was
raging. He proposed to send out an equipped
ship. Many were ready to subscribe, and Jenner
himself offered a thousand pounds ; but there was
delay. In the meantime Dr. De Carro, of Vienna,
had made good use of some lymph received from
Jenner, and had spread the practice through
Austria, Hungary, Poland, and part of Germany.
Lord Elgin, our ambassador at the Porte, who had
heard little of vaccination when in England,
obtained lymph from De Carro for his son, and
vaccination spread rapidly among Europeans in
Constantinople, and then among Mohammedans.

Lord and Lady Elgin, on a tour through the
islands of the Archipelago (during which the Elgin
Marbles were purchased) preached vaccination.
Turks, Greeks, and Armenians were eager for it, and
in Salonika alone 1130 persons were vaccinated.

India was crying out for it. The Governor of
Bombay appealed to Lord Elgin, and received a
quill of lymph in 1801. Lord Elgin afterwards
wrote to the Hon. Arthur Paget : ' I have so many
applications for vaccine virus from Bussora, the

London – Hertford Street
March 30 1803

Dear Sir

Since the commencement of our correspondence, great as my satisfaction has often been in the perusal of your letters, I do not recollect when you have favor'd me with one that has afforded me pleasure equal to the last. The regret I have experienc'd at finding every endeavor to send the Vaccine Virus to India prove abortive is scarcely to be describ'd to you. Judge then what pleasure you convey in assuring me that my wishes are accomplish'd.

I am confident that had not my Opponents in this Country endeavor'd to ridicule my Ideas of the origin of the Disease & been so absurdly clamorous (particularly P. & W.) the Asiatics would

. . . .

Excuse this stupid Letter. I write to you under the Influence of the prevailing Epidemical Catarrh, which doubtless has pervaded the Austrian Dominions —

Adieu my dear Sir — Accept my best wishes & be assured how happy I am in subscribing myself

Your sincere Friend
& faithful humble Serv.
Edw. Jenner

515

Autograph letter by Jenner in the Royal College of Physicians written to Dr. De Carro of Vienna, 1803.

East Indies, and Ceylon, that I beg that you will immediately apply to Dr. De Carro and request him to send some by every courier.'

Fortunately Dr. Sacco of Milan had found vaccine virus among the cows of Lombardy. He wrote to Jenner : ' With this virus there have already been more than eight thousand vaccinations performed with the most happy success. Several hundred of these have been subjected to variolous inoculation, and have resisted it.' Dr. Sacco was able to furnish Dr. De Carro with the lymph required for India. There, Hindoo and Mohammedan physicians eagerly learnt to vaccinate, for smallpox was a curse of India. Hindoos from their veneration for the cow readily accepted the treatment.

The following letter to De Carro (in the College of Physicians) shows Jenner's delight at the advent of vaccine lymph in India.

' London : Hertford Street.
' March 30, 1803.

' Dear Sir,—Since the commencement of our correspondence, great as my satisfaction has often been in the perusal of your letters, I do not recollect when you have favord me with one that has afforded me pleasure equal to the last. The regret I have experienced at finding every endeavor to send the vaccine virus to India prove abortive is scarcely to be described to you. Judge then what pleasure you convey in assuring me that my wishes are accomplished.

'I am confident that had not my opponents in this country endeavord to ridicule my ideas of the origin of the Disease & been so absurdly clamorous (particularly P. & W.) the Asiatics would long since have enjoyed the blessings of vaccination and many a victim been rescued from an untimely grave. However, the decisive experiments of Dr. Loy[1] on this subject have silenced their tongues for ever, and happy am I to see this interesting work translated by you, and I hope in its new dress that it will traverse the world over.

'I do not imagine that a sea voyage conduces to injure the Vaccine Virus, for I have repeatedly sent it to America with all its perfections about it. . . . With respect to its failure in the East Indies when sent from this country, we must, I conceive, attribute it to the length of time, chiefly, that passes away during the voyage;[2] and in some measure to the want of management of it when it arrives, as it must necessarily fall into the hands of those who are inexperienced in the mode of using vaccine matter after it has suffered desiccation. . . .

'I am happy to find an opinion taken up by me, & mentioned in my first publication has so able a supporter as yourself. I thought it highly probable, and still am impressed with the same sentiment, that the small pox might be a malignant variety of the cow-pox. But this idea was scouted by my countrymen, particularly P. & W.

'When I first heard that the Physicians on the Continent were vaccinating sheep with the view of rendering them unsusceptible of the *Rot*, I was astonished; but now I perceive that this arose from a want of due

---

[1] Dr. J. G. Loy, of Whitby, published a pamphlet on vaccination.
[2] Lymph deteriorates on exposure to heat. That may have been the cause of its failure.

precision in language. What we mean by the *Rot* is a disease of the liver . . . occasioned, as we imagine by the sheep's living on marshy land.[1] I have dissected many that have died of it. The rot in Hares (which I also learn from dissection) is precisely the same disease as that in sheep. But the disease you describe is very different . . .

' It affords me pleasure to find that the malevolent attack of Pearson and Woodville on my reputation excites the same indignation on the Continent as, I trust, it does among us.

' I always foresaw that the conduct of the former would require no observations from me. Every sentence he has penned with a view to my injury recoils upon himself. You shall see some pamphlets written in reply to his pamphlet.

' Excuse this stupid letter. I write to you under the influence [2] of the prevailing Epidemical Catarrh, which doubtless has pervaded the Austrian Dominions.

' Adieu my dear Sir,—Accept my best wishes and be assured how happy I am in subscribing myself,

Your sincere friend
& faithful humble serv^{t.}

' Dr. De Carro,   Edw^{D.} JENNER.
    Vienna.'

---

[1] ' Rot ' in sheep is now known to be caused by a parasite which inhabits a water-snail—becomes encysted on wet herbage and when swallowed by sheep or other warm-blooded animals (including man), becomes the ' liver fluke.' Hence watercress should be carefully washed and examined before being placed on the table.

[2] ' Under the influence ' is quite the right expression, for the old Italian physicians thought that epidemic catarrh which, at times, seemed to invade wide districts of the earth at the same moment, could only be due to a ' flowing in '—an influenza—from the planets.

Later, Calcutta and its dependencies thankfully sent Jenner a testimonial of £3000—afterwards increased to £4000; Bombay sent £2000, and Madras £1383. Dr. H. Scott, President of the Medical Board of the Bombay Presidency, who had been active in promoting the testimonial to Jenner, wrote :

'Vaccine inoculation goes on here with its usual success. In this Island, swarming with mankind, no loss has been suffered by the smallpox for several years, since the introduction of the vaccine inoculation.'

Thus vaccination spread through the East.

At this time, at Cheltenham, Jenner had comparative rest from the incessant efforts he had made to correct mistakes, and teach the correct practice of vaccination. While there he offered gratuitous vaccination to all the poor, and numbers of children were brought to him from the town, and from surrounding parishes. One incident delighted him. The inhabitants of a parish, which had long held back, suddenly brought their children. Inquiries were made, and it was found that the parish authorities had ordered vaccination, because ' the cost of coffins for the children who were cut off by smallpox proved burdensome to the parish.'

On the Continent the practice of vaccination spread rapidly. A temple was dedicated to Jenner at Brünn. The Dowager-Empress of Russia wrote him a gracious letter on the service he had rendered to humanity ; and enclosed a valuable diamond ring.[1]

At Copenhagen a Committee, appointed by the King, reported that from the ' most exact observations vaccination . . . at least for a time . . . prevents the contagion of smallpox '—that it is not attended with danger—and recommends that it should be performed gratis at institutions for the poor. Later on Napoleon issued a decree that 100,000 francs should be spent on vaccination in France.

The Royal Society of Göttingen elected Jenner an honorary member. Dr. Davids[2] of Rotterdam, to whom he had sent lymph, wrote : ' The name of Jenner is adored . . . vaccination was introduced just at the moment the smallpox made ravages through the whole country, but, thank God, not one is infected after the vaccine.' Dr. De Carro, who had done so much to promote vaccination throughout Europe, in a letter to a Mr. Ring, said :

' After three years of success I need not tell you what I think of vaccination. . . . Remember me to Dr. Jenner.

[1] ' Its pecuniary value was about £1500. It consisted of a cluster of brilliants, with a very large one in the centre . . . We could never prevail upon its owner to wear it except upon the birthday of one of his children.' *Reminiscences of a Literary Life*, by Rev. T. F. Dibdin, 1836.

[2] Dr. Davids had translated Jenner's pamphlet.

No medical man ever excited my admiration and veneration so much. He is not only great by the magnitude of his discovery, but he is also great by the manner in which he conducted his researches ; by the perfection that he gave to them before he published his work, and by the extreme modesty with which he speaks of himself. His fame increases daily.' [1]

De Carro's estimate of Jenner's character, and of the care taken in his investigations, agreed with that of Dr. Baron.

[1] Baron : *Life of Edward Jenner*, i. 474.

CHAPTER 5

Jenner's personal expenditure on vaccination. Discussion in Parliament and Government grant of £10,000. Success of vaccination in Germany, Vienna, Italy, and Newfoundland. Jenner made honorary associate of the Physical Society, and D.C.L. of Cambridge, U.S.A. Royal Jennerian Society. Pearson's attack on Jenner. Jenner presented with gold medal of Medical Society. Attack on and defence of Jenner. Practises in Mayfair. Return to country life. Vaccinates gratuitously at Cheltenham.

As a missionary of vaccination, Jenner had made no attempt to enrich himself. He had spent much of his private fortune, and he had sacrificed professional advantages. His patience in answering innumerable letters, and in instructing others, was inexhaustible. This was felt so strongly by his neighbours in Gloucestershire that a service of plate was presented to him by a committee of Gloucestershire residents, headed by the Earl of Berkeley.

At the same time it was decided that his claim to a grant should be brought before the House of Commons. A petition to that effect was consequently presented in March 1802. Mr. Addington,[1] the Prime Minister, reported that the King

---

[1] Afterwards Viscount Sidmouth.

strongly recommended the petition to Parliament. It was pointed out that the petitioner had gained nothing by his important discovery, but had been a considerable loser—that he had relinquished prospects of emolument by propagating and extending it, and rendering it of universal utility to the human race, rather than of private advantage to himself.

The petition was referred to a Parliamentary Committee. Admiral Berkeley,[1] the chairman, said that Dr. Jenner's discovery

' is the greatest ever made for the preservation of the human species. It is proved that in these United Kingdoms alone 45,000 persons annually die of smallpox . . . that throughout the world every second a victim is sacrificed at the altar of the most horrible of all disorders. . . . I shall therefore move that a sum of not less than £10,000 be granted ; but when I do this, I declare I do not think it sufficient.'

W. Windham pointed out that Dr. Jenner did not keep his discovery a secret. Had he done so, the House would have been called upon to pay heavily for its purchase. Wilberforce proposed a larger grant, as Jenner had devoted more than twenty years to ' completing the discovery.' Sir

---

[1] Admiral Berkeley (son of the 4th Earl and 17th Baron Berkeley) had the chief command on the Portuguese coast from 1808 to 1812. He was appointed Lord High Admiral of Portugal in acknowledgment of his services to the country.

Everard Home, Sir Walter Farquhar, and Lord Berkeley gave evidence in favour of the grant.

Many witnesses were examined—not only those in favour of vaccination, but also those who opposed it. In a letter to his friend, Mr. Hicks, Jenner wrote :

' April 1802.

' . . . There is a fundamental error, in my opinion, in the conduct of the Committee. Having been put in possession of the laws of vaccination by so great a number of the first medical men in the world—namely, that when properly conducted it never fails, and when improperly, that it will fail—they should not have listened to every blockhead who chose to send up a supposed case of its imperfection ; but this is the plan pursued, and if they do not give it up, they may sit till the end of their lives ; for the vaccinator, like the smallpox inoculator, will go on for ever committing blunders . . . How unjust it is to make me answerable for all the ignorance and carelessness of others.'

Jenner's practice had, no doubt, suffered by his discovery, which involved long visits to London. He narrates how

' Since I first made my discovery public I was compelled to adopt this measure ' (frequent visits to London, etc.) ' from observing the confusion that was arising among practitioners in the Metropolis . . . from misrepresentation of my facts by some, and a careless observance of them by others. Foreign nations, too, were sending deputies to inquire into the new practice,

G

and as my aim was to diffuse the knowledge of it as widely as possible, and as expeditiously, this work, I was confident, could not go on so well by correspondence as by constant personal intercourse. My receipts arising from the practice have gone but a little way in reimbursing me. My private affairs, as my time was so incessantly occupied in establishing the new practice, have, of course, experienced that derangement which neglect always brings on.'

The House of Commons, at last, by a majority of three, voted in favour of a grant of £10,000.

Every post now brought letters from some part of the world. One from America announced that the degree of D.C.L. of Cambridge, Massachusetts, had been conferred on him. He was given the freedom of Edinburgh and of Dublin. Dr. Struve [1] wrote from Saxony :

' Great and honoured Sir,—The practice of Vaccine Inoculation, your discovery, is highly esteemed and cultivated by the Germans, insomuch that not a single town or village can be found in which persons have not been shielded by the Jennerian ægis from the contagion of smallpox.'

The Germans, who had been cautious in accepting smallpox inoculation, were welcoming vaccination. The Austrian Government passed an ordinance recommending it, and smallpox was almost banished

[1] of Gorlitz.

from Vienna. Dr. Sacco, unwearied in his work, wrote to say that 60,000 vaccinations had taken place in the Italian Republic ; and from Newfoundland Jenner's friend, the Rev. J. Clinch, wrote :

' Many opportunities soon offered at St. John's, where smallpox was making great ravages. The inhabitants saw, at first with astonishment, that those who had gone through Jennerian inoculation were exposed to infection without the least inconvenience. . . . It will annihilate the worst and most dreadful of all disorders.'

At a meeting of the Physical Society, held at Guy's Hospital, Jenner was received with ' universal and rapturous applause,' [1] and a new order of merit—' Honorary Associate '—was instituted and conferred on him. A vote of congratulation was sent to him by the Medical Society of London.

Many who were not medical practitioners became expert vaccinators. A Miss Bailey, after vaccinating 2600 poor persons, anxious to detect failures, offered a reward of 5s. to anyone who would produce a case of smallpox occurring among them—only one, and that a case of imperfect vaccination, could be found.

Occasionally the clergy undertook vaccination. A Mr. Finch of St. Helen's, Lancashire, wrote to Jenner : ' A few years ago I was in the habit of

---

[1] Baron : *Life of Edward Jenner*, i. 538.

burying two or three children every evening in the spring and autumn who had died of smallpox, but now the disease has entirely ceased.' Mr. Finch had vaccinated 3000 persons.

Dr. Darwin of Derby, Charles Darwin's grand-father, prophesied :

' Your discovery of preventing the dreadful havoc made among mankind by the smallpox, by introducing into the system so mild a disease, as the vaccine inoculation pro-duces, may in time eradicate the smallpox from all civilised countries. . . . Christening and vaccination of children may be performed on the same day.'

Towards the end of 1802 Jenner received a notice that it was proposed to form a ' Royal Jennerian Society,' and that his help would be wanted. Jenner replied that he welcomed the prospect of an Institution for Gratuitous Vaccina-tion, but he hoped that his presence would not be required in London, and that his friend, Dr. Lettsom, might be allowed to represent him.

A meeting was held. The Lord Mayor pre-sided. The Duke of Bedford stated that he had been requested by the Duke of Clarence to move a vote of thanks to Dr. Jenner for the offer of his assistance. The King and Queen became Patron and Patroness.

The following year Jenner was induced to preside at an annual meeting of the Jennerian Society. Thirteen stations were opened for vaccination, and the deaths from smallpox, which had averaged 2018 during the previous fifty years, fell, in 1804, to 622. Later on, the resident vaccinator was found to have broken the rules laid down for him, and to have introduced dangerous practices. The Council decided that his conduct was irregular, and inconsistent with his duty, and that he should be dismissed. Their recommendation was brought before the General Court, a member of which—a friend of the vaccinator—by paying the expenses of some of the voters, managed to pack the Court and to get a majority of three votes against the resolution of the Council. Further action was rendered unnecessary by the resignation of the vaccinator.

The Jennerian Society gradually came to an end, and its place was taken by the National Vaccine Establishment.

The discussion in Parliament, followed by a vote of £10,000, had not the result Jenner's friends intended ; hostility and jealousy were stirred up by it. London practitioners, too, were not inclined to follow rules laid down by a doctor who lived in a little country town.

Some members of the Jennerian Society,

including Dr. G. Pearson, Physician to St. George's Hospital, who had been a friend of Jenner's, were determined that Jenner should not have the credit of being the 'discoverer' of vaccination. They found a Mr. Benjamin Jesty, owner of a dairy-farm in Dorsetshire, who said that he had, long ago, vaccinated his wife and children. Jesty was therefore asked to come to London as a guest of the Society, sit for his portrait, and accept £15 for travelling expenses, and a pair of gold vaccinating lancets as the first known vaccinator.[1]

The following year, at an anniversary meeting of the Medical Society of London, a gold medal was voted to Jenner. Dr. Lettsom [2] gave the address. Jenner was unable to be present owing to the illness of his wife and eldest son. In a letter to Jenner, Lettsom gives an account of a dinner at which Dr. Pearson stated that Jenner's discovery was 'no discovery,' but a 'rascally ignorant business.' [3] Lettsom pointed out that, although cow-pox had long been found by 'incidental experience a security against smallpox, it had never been applied

---

[1] E. M. Crookshank : *History of Vaccination.*

[2] J. C. Lettsom, M.D., was born on his father's estate on Little Vandyke, one of the many small West Indian Islands—was educated in England, returned to West Indies after the death of father and elder brother, and liberated his slaves. He then practised in Red Lion Square, London. 'The name of Lettsom was to be found associated with every project for the public good.' Munk : *Roll of the Royal College of Physicians,* ii. 288.

[3] Baron : *Life of Edward Jenner,* ii. 32.

to any beneficial purpose till the genius of Jenner discriminated its powers, and introduced it into practice.' Lettsom warmly defended Jenner, showed Pearson's mistakes, and convinced those present that Jenner alone had the right to be styled the ' discoverer ' of scientific vaccination.

A writer in the ' Edinburgh Review ' [1]—evidently Sydney Smith himself—in an article of more than thirty pages, wrote :

' Nor do we believe that the virulence of political animosity, or personal rivalry, or revenge, ever gave rise, among the lowest and most prostituted scribblers, to so much coarseness, illiberality, violence, and absurdity as is here exhibited by gentlemen of sense and education, discussing a point of professional science with a view to the good of mankind.

' At one time we were so overpowered by the rude clamour of the combatants that we were tempted to abandon the task, and leave it to some more athletic critic to collect the facts, and the little reasoning . . . in this tempest of the medical world. We were encouraged, however, to proceed by the excellent pamphlet of Mr. Moore [2] (*A Reply to Anti-vaccinists.*)'

Sydney Smith, in criticising the writings of Dr. Rowley [3] and Dr. Squirrel, says that Squirrel ' leaped from his cage upon the whole herd of vaccinators,' that his book was the ' most entertaining of all,' that ' never was anything so ill-written,

---

[1] *Edinburgh Review*, ix. 63.   [2] *Ibid.*, ix. 90.   [3] *Ibid.*, ix. 82.

or so vulgar and absurd produced before by a person entitling himself a doctor of medicine.' Squirrel had even complained to King George III of the parliamentary grant to Jenner.

Dr. Valentin, of Nancy, a well-known French physician, admirer of Jenner and his work, came to London in 1803. Valentin had shown that it was possible, not only to vaccinate cows and horses, and produce the typical vaccine vesicle, but also goats, donkeys, and sheep. During his visit he brought about peace between Woodville and Jenner, who had made a bitter enemy of Woodville by pointing out that while carrying on vaccination and inoculation together at the smallpox hospital, he had contaminated the vaccine which he had distributed.

Jenner was now a public character. Demands on his time and attention increased, and correspondence became a burden. Mr. Addington (the Prime Minister), and other Members of Parliament, who had supported the vote of £10,000, at length persuaded Jenner that it was his duty to take a house in London ; and so fate compelled one who was more than fifty years of age, and who, from youth upwards, had avoided London, to take the lease of a house in Hertford Street, Mayfair, and begin a London practice.

Jenner was not in his element. He had not

gone through the unconscious education slowly
acquired by those who are compelled to live in
daily contact with groups of fellow-men—equals—
sometimes rivals—and not always friendly ;   a
training which creates that necessary tolerance of
all humanity—conspicuous in the good temper of
a London crowd. His mind had not been inoculated against over-sensitiveness to criticism. Unfair
opposition, the elbowing by those who pushed
themselves forward in order to have their names
connected with a discovery that was not theirs, and
frequent misrepresentations in the Press, disconcerted him.

Patients did not flock to his house in Mayfair.
His work was unremunerative—expenses were
heavy, the grant from the Treasury was delayed
for two years, and then nearly a thousand pounds
was deducted from it for taxes ; so after three
months, the lease of the house and the London
practice were given up, and Jenner found himself
again in the country.

Failures in vaccination were continually being
reported, but Jenner held to his belief that if
properly conducted, vaccination affords the same
protection against smallpox, as that obtained by
inoculation. Although away from London, he
was not idle ; he writes : ' I am at least six hours
daily, with my pen in my hand, bending over

writing paper, till I am grown as crooked as a cow's horn.' He had become, as he said, ' vaccine clerk to the world.'

At Cheltenham he vaccinated gratuitously ' all who came. Sometimes he had nearly three hundred persons at his door.' [1] One instance of the efficacy of vaccination delighted him. A poor widow and her children were under the same roof with a labourer who had caught smallpox. She had resigned herself to her fate, when a neighbour persuaded her to go to Cheltenham and consult Jenner. He was away, but the manservant, who had been with him many years, found someone with an ' eighth day ' vaccinated arm, and from it vaccinated the whole group. The result was that they all escaped smallpox, except one child who had a mild attack. Jenner had long ago discovered that vaccination three days after exposure to smallpox was a protection, but this family had been in the same small house with the sick labourer for nearly *five* days.

In a letter from Cheltenham to a friend he writes:

' I hope you are well and happy—and so does my dear Mrs. Jenner who, thank God, has gone on better than I expected. As for myself I bear the fatigues and worries of a public character better, by far, than those,

[1] Baron : *Life of Edward Jenner,* ii. 53.

who know the acuteness of my feelings, could have anticipated. Happy should I be to give up my laurels for the repose of retirement, did I not feel it my duty to be in the world. I certainly derive the most soothing consolation from my labours. . . .

' Cheltenham is much improved since you saw it. It is too gay for me. I still like my rustic haunt, old Berkeley, best ; where we are all going in about a fortnight. Edward is growing tall, and has long looked over my head. Catherine, now eleven years old, is a promising girl, and Robert, eight years old, is just a chip of the old block.'

CHAPTER 6

Influence of Jenner in Europe. Napoleon, Emperor of Austria, and King of Spain release prisoners at his request. Anti-vaccinists report that vaccinated children have the faces of cows. The Royal College of Physicians reports favourably on vaccination. Parliamentary vote of £20,000 to Jenner. Sir Lucas Pepys. Plans for a National Vaccine Establishment drawn up by Jenner. Refuses nominal directorship. Death of eldest son. Case of Lord Grosvenor's son. Jenner elected Associate of the National Institute of France. Letter from S. T. Coleridge.

VACCINATION was rapidly spreading and smallpox diminishing throughout the world ; but in England the movement was slow. In a letter to Mr. Dunning, dated December 23, 1804, Jenner writes :

' . . . Foreigners hear with the utmost astonishment, that in some parts of England there are persons who still inoculate for smallpox. It must, indeed, excite their wonder when they see that disease in some of their largest cities, and in wide-extended districts around them, totally exterminated.

' Let us not, my friend, vex ourselves too much at what we see here ; let us consider this but a speck, when compared with the wide surface of our planet, over which, thank God, vaccine has shed her influence. From the potentate to the peasant, in every country, but this, she is received with " grateful and open arms." '

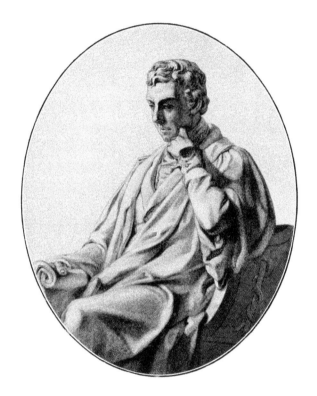

EDWARD JENNER

Bronze statue by W. C. Marshall, R.A., erected in Trafalgar Square, A.D. 1858.
The statue was removed to Kensington Gardens four years later.

(From an engraving by J. Brown.)

With foreign nations at this time, Jenner's name had extraordinary power. Even Napoleon, at war with England, was ready to grant Jenner's requests. Among Englishmen detained in France at the end of the short-lived Treaty of Amiens were Dr. Wickham (an Oxford travelling-fellow) and a Mr. Williams. Both were suffering from confinement. Jenner applied to the Committee of Vaccination in Paris for their release. The Committee suggested a letter to Napoleon. This was written, and the men were allowed to go their way. Napoleon is reported to have said : ' Jenner ! Ah, we can refuse nothing to that man.'

An adventurous young Canadian, W. D. Powell (son of the Chief Justice of the Court of the King's Bench in Upper Canada), had been captured on board Miranda's squadron [1] by the Spanish Navy. He was tried and sentenced to ten years' confinement, with hard labour. Jenner appealed to the King of Spain. He regretted that the petition could not be presented through an ambassador, but he was encouraged to hope, from the magnanimity shown by His Majesty in the glorious expedition to disseminate vaccination throughout the world—to friend and foe alike—that the petition might be granted. The result was that young Powell was

[1] Francesco Miranda, a Spanish-American, following the example of North America, began the revolt of South America against Spain.

allowed to return to his relations in Canada. He wrote a warm letter of thanks to Jenner.

On another occasion a petition was sent by Jenner to the Emperor of Austria, begging for a passport for a Mr. Sinclair, who was detained in Vienna. This was granted ; and two other Englishmen were liberated on Jenner's appealing to Napoleon through the Emperor's physician, Baron Corvisart. In return Baron Corvisart asked Jenner to use his influence with the British Government in order to obtain the release of a young friend. Jenner at first tried in vain. His request was eventually granted.

Abroad, Englishmen whose business had nothing to do with the war travelled with passports signed by Jenner, such as :

' I hereby certify that Mr.——, the bearer of this, who is about to sail on board the —— has no other object in view than the recovery of his health.

EDWARD JENNER.'

If the ship was captured by a French privateer, the bearer would be well treated, and probably given his liberty.

In May 1806 Jenner was elected a Fellow of the Royal College of Physicians of Edinburgh.

The following July the subject of vaccination, smallpox inoculation, and remuneration to Jenner, again came before the House of Commons. Lord Henry Petty (afterwards Lord Lansdowne) proposed [1] that the College of Physicians be requested

' to enquire into the progress of vaccination, and to assign the causes of its success having been retarded throughout the United Kingdom ; in order that their report may be made, . . . and that we may take the most proper means of publishing it to the inhabitants at large . . . If the result of such proposed enquiry turns out a corroboration of the beneficial effects, which other nations seem convinced are derived from vaccination . . . it will prove that the bad effects which have been ascribed to vaccination have been dreadfully exaggerated ; and that the temporary duration of its benefits in a few cases has been owing to some kind of mismanagement.'

Inoculation, Baron reports, had been

' abandoned by almost every respectable medical man . . . but it had been taken up by a set of unprincipled and ignorant persons. These, reckless of the miseries they spread abroad, extort from the prejudiced parent a pittance sufficient to excite their cupidity.'

But it was by no means an easy task to make inoculation illegal. The Duke of Bedford, Lord-Lieutenant of Ireland, wrote to Jenner from Dublin :

'. . . Any testimony, however sanctioned by the College of Physicians, or by Parliament, will I fear, have

---

[1] Baron : *Life of Edward Jenner*, ii. 157.

but little weight in convincing the obstinate, the interested, or the prejudiced. Some legislative restraint must be adopted against that pernicious and fatal error, which permits a man, with impunity, to spread the contagion of a loathsome and cruel disorder around his neighbourhood, and to carry the seeds of disease and death through the streets of the metropolis.'

'These suggestions,' Baron continues, 'were not relished by the House. Just and moderate though they were, they seemed to have too much the aspect of compulsion ; and the liberty of doing wrong was still left among the privileges of free-born Englishmen,' and so smallpox inoculation remained legal long after Jenner's time.[1]

Opposition by the anti-vaccinists went on. A Dr. William Rowly, of Oxford, who ought to have known better, published and distributed a *Solemn Appeal against Vaccination*, with illustrations of vaccinated children becoming, in form and feature, like cows. It increased the prejudice against vaccination, and brought about disgusting abuse of Jenner. Jenner, too, was accused of dishonesty, because he had inoculated his son. The boy had been in contact with smallpox : no lymph for vaccination was available ; a previous vaccination, performed long ago, had given uncertain results ; so inoculation became a necessary precaution.

---

[1] Inoculation was made illegal in 1840.

Meanwhile, in the House of Commons, Lord Henry Petty's motion was carried. The College of Physicians ably performed the duty imposed on it, and collected evidence, which proved to be strongly in favour of vaccination. Spencer Perceval,[1] Chancellor of the Exchequer, then moved (July 1807) that a grant of £10,000 be allowed to Jenner for his discovery, and for the fact that he had presented it to the world. After some discussion £20,000 was voted—60 for and 47 against the motion.

In an interview with Spencer Perceval Jenner complained of the reckless and 'licentious' manner in which smallpox inoculation was being conducted in London :

' I instanced,' he says, ' the mortality it occasioned in language as forcible as I could utter, and showed him clearly that it was the great source from which this pest was disseminated through the country as well as through the town. But alas ! all I said availed nothing ; and the speckled monster is still to have the liberty that the smallpox hospital . . . the delusions of Moseley,[2] and the caprices and prejudices of the misguided poor can possibly give him. I cannot express the disappointment I felt at this interview.'

In 1808, Parliament decided that there should

---

[1] Five years afterwards that able statesman was assassinated in the lobby of the House of Commons.

[2] Dr. Moseley, Physician to Chelsea Hospital, published reports that vaccinated children grew to resemble cattle in form and feature.

H

be a great National Vaccine Establishment for gratuitous vaccination and supply of lymph. Sir Lucas Pepys, then President of the Royal College of Physicians, was requested to organise it. Dr. Munk, the College biographer,[1] says that Pepys was a man of ' great firmness and determination,' inclined to be ' dictatorial.' He was Physician-in-Ordinary to George III. In a lately published diary of Robert Greville,[2] the King, at Kew, is described as pointing to the strait-waistcoat[3] he was wearing, and making a pitiful appeal for release to Sir Lucas Pepys.

Pepys became Physician-General to the Army, and confined his appointments of physicians to the Army to those who had diplomas of the College of Physicians, thus excluding many who had seen previous service in the Army—a custom he was compelled to abandon.

Jenner, when asked by Pepys to draw up plans and an estimate of expenses for the Vaccine Establishment, assented willingly. He remained five months in London, helping in its organisation. He was then recalled to Berkeley by the serious illness of his children.

While at Berkeley he learnt that the Board of

---

[1] W. Munk, M.D. : *Roll of the Royal College of Physicians*, 2nd edition, 1878, ii. 306.

[2] Bladon : *Diaries of Robert Greville*.

[3] A waistcoat made of strong material, with long sleeves fastened together at the back, formerly used to restrain violent lunatics.

the National Vaccine Establishment, which consisted of the President and four Censors of the Royal College of Physicians, and the Master and two Wardens of the Royal College of Surgeons, had rejected most of the names of those recommended by him as eminently qualified to be officers of the vaccinating stations—that he was to be styled ' Director,' but to have no voice in the management. The village doctor could not be allowed a seat on the Board.

Jenner naturally refused to be nominal Director of an Institution he could have no part in directing ; but, although hurt at the ruling of the Board, he was ready to help with advice wherever it was wanted.

This exclusion of the discoverer of vaccination from the Board of the National Vaccine Establishment seems incredibly mean. Not only had Pepys learnt all he knew of vaccination from Jenner, but he had requested Jenner to vaccinate a member of his own family. In a letter, written two years before, Jenner says :

' I have just received a note from the President of the College of Physicians, Sir Lucas Pepys, requesting me to vaccinate his grandson. Two years ago the worthy President would as soon have had the boy's skin touched with the fang of a viper as the vaccine lancet.'

So Jenner would have nothing to do officially with the Vaccine Establishment.   Lord Somerville,[1]

[1] President of the Board of Agriculture.

who had warmly supported the Government grant, wrote to him :

'. . . You keep aloof in this new Vaccine National Establishment, and wise you are in doing it, for well I know that the mean spirit, which presides sometimes, of jealousy and intrigue, is hostile to your nature ; and you are now enabled to keep a whip ready for the backs of those who play foul in it.   In this way you will be of twice the use you could otherwise be . . . When you come to town you owe me a visit at this farm, which for purity of air, and beauty of views, can hardly be equalled.

Ever yours sincerely, My dear Sir,

I am, Yours,

SOMERVILLE.

'Fair-Mile Farm,
Cobham, Surrey.'

The year 1810 brought sorrow to Jenner.   His eldest son, Edward, always a delicate boy, died, and he also lost his friend and patient, Lord Berkeley.   Although the boy's death had long been expected, it came a crushing blow to the father.   He wrote to his friend, John Ring :

' One would suppose that the mind would become in some measure reconciled to an event, however melancholy, that one knows to be inevitable, when it has made such gradual approaches ; but I know, from sad experience, that the edge of sensibility is not thus to be blunted.'

But sorrow had the effect of deadening Jenner's sensitiveness to attacks in the Press.   He writes :

'Whether it be from age, long retirement, or what, I cannot tell, but somehow or other, I feel myself less disposed to notice the malevolence of my enemies.'

The shock of his son's death seriously affected his health. He found himself unable to perform the ordinary duties of life, and so, by the advice of medical friends, he moved to Bath and underwent the severe medical treatment of that date. After a time he appears again at Cheltenham, broken in health, but continuing his work.

The following year an unfortunate event was made the most of by the anti-vaccinists. A son of Lord Grosvenor, who had been vaccinated ten years before by Jenner himself, had an attack of confluent smallpox. Out of the thousands who had been vaccinated by Jenner, not one had hitherto been known to have contracted smallpox ; but the importance of this patient roused popular clamour against vaccination, and Jenner was worried by it.

The child had been delicate. Jenner, against his own principles, had been persuaded by the mother to vaccinate in one place only, and that had been rubbed by the nurse.

Jenner was troubled too by another matter. He was requested to give evidence before the House of Lords on the Berkeley peerage. Nervous and over-sensitive, he dreaded mental breakdown. Fortunately dissolution of Parliament saved him from being forced into a position which all family physicians in the confidence of their patients would, if possible, avoid.[1]   He said :

'I can compare my feelings to those of no one but Cooper the poet, when his intellect at last gave way to his fears about the execution of his office in the House of Lords.   It was reading " Cooper's Life," I believe, which saved my own senses, by putting me fully in view of my danger.   For many weeks before the meeting I began to be agitated, and, as it approached, I was actually deprived of both appetite and sleep ; . . . the meeting was at length interrupted by a dissolution of Parliament . . . to my no small delight.'

At the same time he was cheered by receiving a warm letter from Sir Joseph Banks announcing that the National Institute of France had elected him an Associate, and congratulating him on ' obtaining a place among a body of men who have so little humbled themselves before the arbitrary dispositions of their Sovereign, as to have retained the title of National when that of Imperial [2] was offered to them ' by Napoleon.   It was some consolation to receive congratulations from the President of the Royal Society, which had been unwilling to accept his paper on vaccination.

S. T. Coleridge too—full of admiration for the discoverer of vaccination—sent Jenner a long letter written with the poet's accustomed fluency :

[1] The question of the Berkeley peerage was referred to a committee.
[2] The word ' Imperial ' was afterwards adopted.

'7 Portland Place, Hammersmith,
27 Sept. 1811.

' Dear Sir,—I take the liberty of intruding on your time first to ask you where, and in what publication, I shall find the fullest history of the vaccine matter as a preventive of smallpox. I mean the year in which the thought first suggested itself to you (and surely no honest heart would suspect me of flattery if I had said *inspired* into you by the All-preserver, as a counterpoise to the crushing weight of this unexampled war), and the progress of its realisation to the present day. . . . I have planned a poem on this theme, which, after long deliberation, I have convinced myself is capable in the highest degree of being poetically treated according to our divine bard's own definition of poetry . . .

Most sincerely your respectful friend
and servant,
S. T. COLERIDGE.'

There seems to be no record of the answer. The reply could not have been an encouraging one, for in a letter dated 1813 [1] he modestly writes :

' An old associate of mine has long been threatening to send some memoir into the world, but I have been constantly intreating him to desist, conceiving that, independently of the vaccine discovery, there was nothing of sufficient interest to engage the attention of the public.'

Jenner probably sent a like answer to Coleridge ; and thus the world lost a poem which would have been historic.

[1] Baron : *Life of Edward Jenner*, ii. 387.

CHAPTER 7

National Vaccine Establishment. Sir John Moore's death. Jenner
corresponds with James Moore. Vaccine lymph from horses. Satisfactory reports from Havana, South America, Milan, Vienna, Russia,
Denmark, India, and Java. Sir A. Crichton on vaccination in Russia.
Oxford confers degree of M.D. on Jenner. Personal assurances of
success of vaccination from Emperor of Russia, King of Prussia, and
Blücher. Honour from Munich. Death of invalid wife. Jenner
retires to Berkeley. His character. Notes from *Annals of Medical
History*.

In 1812 Jenner was at Berkeley, cheered by the
year's Report of the National Vaccine Establishment. That institution was now under the
direction of James Moore,[1] who, like his brother,
Sir John (lately killed while defending our troops
during their hurried embarkation at Corunna
and mourned by all his men) was a man of attractive
character; and of better understanding than many
of those who were engaged in the dispute on
vaccination.

Jenner and James Moore were firm friends, and
Jenner was always ready to put his experience at
the service of the Institution which had refused

---

[1] Author of *A History of Smallpox*, and of a *Life of Sir John Moore*.

him a place on its Board. He had written to Moore a month after Sir John Moore's death, on the care required for successful vaccination :

' I recommend extreme deliberation in framing this important document ' (rules for the Institution). ' As for yourself, my dear friend, it cannot be expected that you can at present coolly exercise your judgment on anything of the kind. . . . Though not as a matter of duty . . . , yet be assured I shall always be ready, as an act of courtesy, to do anything in my power to promote the ends for which the Government Institution was founded.'

For years Jenner continued to do this.

Something in James Moore's character, as in that of his brother, disarmed hostility. Even his opponent, John Birch, Surgeon to St. Thomas's Hospital, when writing against those who wished to replace inoculation by vaccination—a practice he considered ' unnatural and unsafe '—could not help speaking of James Moore as ' the ablest and most candid writer that has appeared in support of vaccination ' . . . deserving ' praise for the pleasant manner in which he has treated the subject, but much more for the candour he has shown.'

So, although remaining deaf to Moore's entreaties that he should not remain aloof from the National Vaccine Establishment, Jenner continued to correspond with him, and to supply any information required on the subject uppermost in the minds of both.

He writes to Moore :

' Vaccination at its commencement fell into the hands of many who knew little more about it than its mere outline. One grand error, that was almost universal at that time, was making one puncture only, and consequently one vesicle. . . . I have taken a world of pains to correct this abuse, but still to my knowledge it is going on, and particularly among the faculty in town.'

Evidently Moore is frank with his friend, for Jenner writes to him :

' You don't like my style when I write for the public eye. Nor do I ; but I cannot mend it, for I write then under the impression of fear . . . and when I write in London my brain is full of smoke.'

Jenner always found difficulty in putting his observations and his thoughts into smooth English sentences. His language was apt to become too figurative. He had written in 1809 to the Rev. Dr. Worthington :

' I am by accident become a public character ; and having the worst head for arrangement that was ever placed on man's shoulders, I think myself the most unfit for it. You may form some judgment of my accumulated vexations, when I tell you that I am, at this moment, more than a hundred letters behindhand with my correspondents. I have lately been deprived of the aid of my secretary. He was cut off by the same dreadful disease, which I fear will shortly take my son from me. What dreadful strides pulmonary consumption seems to be making over every part of our island.'

The 'secretary,' a boy in feeble health, but intelligent beyond his years, had lost his father, a poor watchmaker. Jenner—always ready to help less fortunate neighbours—took the lad into the house and made him his secretary, and tutor to his son. Baron writes :

'This extraordinary boy became an inmate of Dr. Jenner's family in 1806, having not then completed his sixteenth year. He was endowed with a singular maturity of judgments, an uncommon delicacy of perception, a quick and vivid imagination, a love of high and enobling thoughts . . . In the space of a few years he had crowded the experience of a lifetime . . . He lived for three years with Jenner and died from pulmonary tubercle in 1809.'

Later on Jenner seems to have realised that pulmonary tubercle can be infectious, for among some notes made by him, and published in the *Annals of Medical History*, is one, dated April 1821, in which he says : 'Pulmonary consumption is certainly contagious ; but less so than any disease I know that is contagious.'

The close atmosphere of sick rooms of that day not only hindered the recovery of those suffering from pulmonary tubercle, but was liable to spread the infection to others. Jenner, by his own observation and unhappy experience, arrived at a truth which took the medical profession another fifty years to learn.

Among his letters to Moore is one in which Jenner shows that horses as well as cows apparently transmit vaccine virus. He writes :

'. . . Great numbers of young carters, in the course of my practice here have come to me from the hills to be vaccinated ; but the average number which resisted has been one half. On inquiry, many of them have recollected having sores on their hands and fingers from dressing horses affected with sore heels, and being so ill as to be disabled from following their work ; and on several of their hands, I have found a cicatrix as perfect and as characteristically marked as if it had arisen from my own vaccination.'

Jenner at first believed that horses were the origin of cow-pox in dairies, for horses and cows were affected at the same time, in the same districts. No doubt carters, who milked cows after dressing horses' heels, often carried the infection to cows. Later, Jenner learnt that horses were not the only source of infection ; also that there were other causes of sore heels, for no part of the body is exposed to such rough usage. Towards the end of his life he made much use of lymph obtained from horses.

And now came a satisfactory year's Report[1] of the National Vaccine Establishment, drawn up under Moore's direction. It recorded that in Havana, where smallpox had been extremely fatal, it had caused no death for two years—that in Spanish America it had been ' extinguished '— that the ' same results were obtained both at Milan and at Vienna . . . where the average mortality from smallpox had amounted to 800 annually '— that in France, out of 2,671,662 persons vaccinated, only 7 had taken smallpox—that in Russia, 1,235,597 had been vaccinated in eight years.

How many millions had been vaccinated in both Old and New Worlds in the few years that had passed since Jenner published the first edition of his pamphlet, it is impossible to estimate.

A letter from Sir Alexander Crichton gives a very interesting account of vaccination in Russia.

Dr. Alexander Crichton, Physician to the Westminster Hospital, became in 1804 Physician in Ordinary to the Emperor Alexander I of Russia. Possibly the Emperor thought the doctor's Christian name a good omen. At all events, Crichton gained the confidence of the Emperor, and became, as his letter to Jenner shows, head of the whole civil medical department of Russia. The Dowager-Empress consulted him on the formation

[1] Baron : *Life of Edward Jenner*, ii. 182.

of her charitable institutions. When he returned to England, George IV knighted him, in the Pavilion at Brighton.

Crichton writes to Jenner : [1]

'St. Petersburg, 12 Sept. 1812.

' Dear Sir,—The re-establishment of peace between England and Russia being happily concluded, I embrace an early opportunity of sending you a letter on the state of vaccination in this Empire. . . . As all the reports on this subject, and indeed all those which regard every branch of Medical Police . . . are addressed to me, it is in my power to give you the most accurate account of the progress of your beneficial discovery. . . . I have annexed a list of all the children who have been vaccinated in the Russian Empire between 1804 and 1812. . . . To show you the manner in which the evidence is collected I have added one of the half-yearly lists of one of the Governments, translated by one of my secretaries into French. I have chosen one of the most distant for this purpose. It is inhabited by different tribes of Tartars. . . . You will find that one of your most zealous vaccinators in these distant regions is a priest of the Great Lama, himself a Lama.

' The whole number of children vaccinated in the Empire amounts to 1,235,597. Now, supposing according to a well-founded rule of calculation, that before the introduction of vaccination, every seventh child died, annually, of smallpox,[2] vaccination has saved the lives of 167,514 children in this Empire.'

[1] Baron : *Life of Edward Jenner*, ii. 183–87.
[2] Moore : *A History of Smallpox*, p. 286.

Crichton also gives a list of the Orders issued by the Emperor.

'. . . All the clergy are to co-operate with the beneficent views of the Emperor . . . A committee of vaccination is to be established in each town . . . The Committees are ordered to see that the practice and art of vaccination be introduced into all schools, and that the *students of all classes be able to practise it before they leave the seminaries, and to see that all midwives be properly instructed in this art* (!)

'. . . The said committees are to distribute a popular work on vaccination printed in all the languages in use throughout the Empire, containing a clear history of the disease—its real signs, with rules when to take the matter to inoculate, and treat the inflammation when accidentally increased.

'Three years to be allowed for vaccinating the whole Empire ; after which period there must not be found one man, woman, or child, who has not been vaccinated.'

But it was not all smooth sailing. Crichton concludes :

'. . . Notwithstanding the order of his Imperial Majesty . . . we find that powerful as his Majesty is . . . there is a power greater than sovereignty, namely, the conscience . . . of men, and in one of the distant governments there exists a peculiar religious sect belonging to the Greek Church, who esteem it a damnable crime to encourage the propagation of any disease, or to employ any doctors or to swallow any medicines. . . . The government have come to the wise resolution of leaving this dispute to time.

Dear Sir, Yours very sincerely,

ALEX. CRICHTON.'

The Government of Russia was then enlightened and tolerant, and the Emperor full of schemes for the good of his subjects, and for a peaceable confederation of nations.

Sir Alexander Crichton's position seems an extraordinary one. Napoleon, five years before (in 1807), had induced Russia to join France against England ; and yet, while Russia is at war with us, a physician to the Westminster Hospital acts as Minister of Health in Russia, with powers over the Russian people far greater than those exercised over Englishmen by any Medical Officer of Health in England.

Relations between nations seem to have been less embittered by war, and international jealousies less active than now. Soult, the French commander, admires and erects a monument to his opponent, James Moore's brother, killed at Corunna. Napoleon, and the Emperor of Austria, and the King of Spain, are all prepared to liberate English subjects, prisoners of war, on a petition from an English doctor. The relentless, uncompromising spirit of modern warfare had not yet arisen.

Far away, in another distant corner of the world, a meeting was held by North American Indians, at which they said :

' We shall not fail to teach our children to speak the name of Jenner, and to thank the Great Spirit, for bestowing upon him so much wisdom, and so much benevolence. We send with this a belt, and a string of Wampum [1] in token of our acceptance of your precious gift ; and we beseech the Great Spirit to take care of you in this world and in the land of Spirits.'

In Denmark 9728 persons are recorded as having died of smallpox between the years 1762 and 1792. Vaccination was introduced about 1802. In 1810 vaccination, by command of the King, was universally adopted and smallpox inoculation was prohibited. From the year 1810 to 1819 not a single case of smallpox occurred.[2] From Sweden, where there had been the same satisfactory results,[3] Jenner received the warmest letter of thanks.

Reports received from Bombay and Bengal showed that vaccination had been carried out in India with good results. In a letter to R. Dunning (1888) [4] Jenner says :

' I have just received the Annual Report from Dr. McKenzie, Superintendent-General of vaccination at

[1] Wampum—cowrie shells, long used by North American tribes (and many early nations) as money. When strung and sewn in patterns on a belt they record pacts and friendship.
[2] Baron : *Life of Edward Jenner*, ii. 446.   [3] *Ibid.*, ii. 253.   [4] *Ibid.*, ii. 359.

Madras. Wonderful to relate, the numbers vaccinated at that Presidency in the course of the last year, amount to 243,175.

' From Bombay I learn the smallpox there is completely subdued, not a single case having occurred for the last two years. All my foreign reports correspond with these.'

These excellent results in Bombay could not be expected to continue for ever. Lady West, the wife of Sir Edward West, first Chief Justice of the King's Court of Bombay, writes in her diary : [1]

' 29 March, 1825.—We have two poor hamauls very ill with smallpox. We have sent them to the native hospital, and I hope they may recover. The cook's mate, a Portuguese, has it, also a horse-keeper. They were vaccinated ; but I suppose it was badly done. So many are now ill who fancied they were safe, that I believe they will not be persuaded to have it done to their children.'

The vaccinator may have carelessly exposed his lymph to an Indian sun.

Sir Stamford Raffles, the able Lieutenant-Governor of Java, who had regenerated the island, appointed vaccinators, under European surgeons, for each district. Later on, he paid a visit to Berkeley. Jenner and the founder of the 'London Zoo' must have had much in common.

In December 1813, Jenner, accompanied by

[1] F. Dawtrey Drewitt : *Bombay in the Days of George IV*, 1907, p. 167.

Dr. Baron, left for Oxford, to receive an honorary M.D. degree at the University. Sir C. Pegge, the Reader in Anatomy, informed him that the degree had been voted unanimously. Efforts were then made by Jenner's friends to induce the Royal College of Physicians to admit him a Fellow, but they were told that this was impossible, unless he passed the usual examinations in Latin. That, Jenner said, he would not do, even for the whole of John Hunter's Museum.

In 1814 Napoleon abdicated, and the allied sovereigns came to England. The cultivated Grand Duchess of Oldenburg, the Emperor of Russia's sister, had several interviews with Jenner, and surprised him by her knowledge of natural history and medicine. Later on the Emperor Alexander himself, in a long interview, told Jenner that his vaccine had nearly subdued smallpox throughout Russia, and congratulated him on the 'delightful feelings' he must experience in having rendered such service to mankind.

The Emperor, who, the evening before, had been entertained at a civic feast, remarked that the English custom of sitting for hours in the 'same room in which you have been eating, must be injurious.' Jenner explained that happily it was not a common custom. Both Emperor and Grand Duchess spoke English fluently.

Jenner also had interviews with the King of Prussia, and with Blücher, both of whom acknowledged that the world was under obligations to him. He received pressing invitations to Berlin. Vaccination had been carried out so efficiently in Prussia that smallpox was almost unknown,[1] and the anniversary of the vaccination of the boy Phipps was kept as a national festival.

From Munich he received the following letter, written in English :

'Munich, Nov. 1, 1814.

' Dear Sir,—I have the honour of presenting to you the Diploma of our Royal Academy of Sciences, as a due acknowledgment of the superiority of that salutiferous genius, by whose infinite merit mankind stands delivered for ever from the most hideous and dreadful of all diseases. Bavaria can boast of being the country in which your glorious discovery found the highest applause. . . . May the blessings of so many millions whose lives you saved, or whose deformities you prevented, contribute to exhilarate the days of their benefactor.

I am, dear Sir, with profoundest veneration,
Your obedient and humble servant,
Dr. S. T. VON SOEMMERING.'

A scheme was then initiated by some of the ladies of England, including Queen Charlotte, to present a testimonial to Jenner.

[1] The same efficiency continued. The average number of deaths from smallpox in Germany for five years—1893–97—was one per million of inhabitants. Edwardes : *Smallpox in Europe*, 1902.

Baron writes of this proposal :

' Mothers whose offspring had been protected . . . daughters whose beauty had been preserved . . . intended to unite in offering a tribute of their gratitude to the author of vaccination. . . . They remembered the anxieties and perils connected with the progress of smallpox, in whatever form it was communicated. Protracted suffering, hideous deformity, shocking to the patient, frightful to the beholder, often terminated by death, or by permanent injury, blasting a mother's fondest hopes ; these, and greater evils, more or less embittered the happiness of every family before the adoption of vaccination.'

These good intentions were not carried out ; all were impoverished owing to the long war.

Jenner was now spending most of his time at Cheltenham, where his wife, over whom he watched with devoted care, was dying of pulmonary tubercle.

In early life much of Mrs. Jenner's time had been devoted to teaching in the Berkeley Sunday School, which had been founded by her. Baron hints that her cheerful resignation in illness, and her devout religious life, influenced her husband, and increased his readiness to forgive those who slandered him.

In 1815 Mrs. Jenner died. It was a heavy blow. Jenner retired, as much as was possible, from public life, and never again, except for a day or two, left his home at Berkeley.

He was haunted by the fear that want of care and the ' extreme ignorance of medical men ' on vaccination, ' will destroy the advantages which the world ought to derive from the practice.' It also became evident that the protecting power of vaccination, as that of inoculation, was liable to wear out after some years, and that revaccination was necessary. This gave those who were opposed both to Jenner and to vaccination an opportunity for attack ; but Jenner had for many years claimed that vaccination only gave the same security as that given by inoculation, or recovery from an attack of smallpox. He gives a case of a woman in his neighbourhood who had smallpox as a child, was a smallpox nurse for years, and eventually died of it. Baron reports :

' He knew that his researches had been conducted with perfect fairness, . . . and that a desire to render his knowledge a source of advantage to his fellow creatures guided all his actions.'

So Jenner turned his back on the world into which fate had thrown him. It is evident that at times he found it difficult to be tolerant to opponents. Overworked and worried, in surroundings to which he was not accustomed, he must occasionally have shown, as many men would, signs of irritation and quick temper. The missionary of vaccination became a crusader. But those who knew him well loved him. Dibdin wrote : ' I never knew a man of a simpler mind, or of a warmer heart, than Dr. Jenner.' [1]

Baron [2] says that he

'was not only humble in all that concerned the greatest incident of his life, he continued so after success had crowned his labours, and after applause, greater than most men can bear, had been bestowed upon him. . . . This was conspicuous when he was living in familiar intercourse with the inhabitants of his native village. If the reader could, in imagination, accompany me, with him, to the dwellings of the poor, and see him kindly and heartily inquiring into their wants, and entering into all the little details of their domestic economy ; or if he could have witnessed him listening with perfect patience and good humour, to the history of their maladies, he would have seen an engaging instance of untiring bene-volence. He was never unwilling to receive anyone, how-ever unseasonable the time may have been. Such were his habits even to the latest period of his life. . . . In the active, and unostentatious exercise of kindness and charity he spent his days. . . . He had a deeply religious mind . . . there was a happy union of seriousness and playfulness, never misplaced. . .

'At first sight his appearance was not very striking. . . . The first things that a stranger would remark were the gentleness, the simplicity, the artlessness of his manner. There was a total absence of all ostentation or

---

[1] T. F. Dibdin : *Reminiscences of a Literary Life*, 1836, p. 199.
[2] Baron : *Life of Edward Jenner*, ii. 299.

display ; so much so that in ordinary intercourse of society he appeared as a person who had no claims to notice. He was perfectly unreserved, and free from all guile. He carried his heart and his mind so openly, that all might read them.'

Some notes which Jenner jotted down in the pocket book he carried with him have lately appeared in *Annals of Medical History*, published in New York. They contain extracts from public speeches, writings of favourite authors, and moral reflections, maxims, medical notes, observations, and passing thoughts—and a list of annual subscriptions to dispensaries and other charities—memoranda all jumbled together, for his own use. They seem to bring us closer to the man. These are some of them :

' The great book of the world is open to all eyes ; my wish is that every human being might be taught to read it. The poor man does not know what a rich library he is in possession of.'

' Steam is the best thing to kill the red spider.'

' When a man becomes a monk he is a mere barrel-organ set to psalm tunes.'

' A herd of cows, when feeding quietly in a meadow, make their slow advance with their heads turned *from* the wind. This appears to be instinctive, to prevent their natural enemies (wolves for example) from approaching unawares—for they (the cows) are quick scented.'

' A medical man, from the nature of things, is always

groping like a miner in the dark without the benefit of a safety lamp.'

'There would be no quacks if physicians had yet learned how to cure diseases.'

'Among the vulgar—the great and the little vulgar—nothing is recorded of vaccination but its imperfections. Its benefits pass by and are forgotten.'

'The student of geology scarcely passes the threshold of his enquiry before he finds himself in a bewildered country. The Mosaic account of the deluge on one side, and the order in which he finds the *mineral cabinets* arranged by the hand of nature on the other.'

'In order to facilitate the enquiry into the cause of the fatal tendency of pulmonary complaints at the present time we should enquire into the habits of our forefathers with regard to their mode of living and exposure to cold air.'

In these last two reflections he was in advance of his generation.

Jenner, as has already been mentioned, was at heart a naturalist—an observant and thoughtful one. Natural history was to him, as it has been to others, a comfort in solitary old age. Linnæus' words, spoken in his last lecture given at the University of Upsala, were true when he said that 'the delights of the pursuit of natural history are not like the ordinary and perishable enjoyments of life, but on the contrary one of the most permanent sources of pleasure which the kindness of providence has opened to the human mind.'

He was, at times, busy preparing (in rather too flowery language !) his paper for the Royal Society on the 'Migration of Birds.' His friend, Henry Shrapnell, helped him in labelling his many specimens of natural history and fossils ; and William Buckland—destined one day to become the first President of the British Association for the Advancement of Science—and also Dean of Westminster— paid him many visits, explored with him the trap rocks at Micklewood, and used his fossil-hammer on the corals at Woodford.

The two naturalists had much in common. Baron says of Jenner :

' In the country where his guests were generally his own immediate connections or intimate friends, the originality of his character came out in the most engaging manner. He almost always brought some intellectual offering to the morning repast. A new fact in natural history, a fossil, or some of the results of his meditations supplied materials for conversation . . . his mirth and gaiety, except when under the pressure of domestic calamity or bodily illness, never long forsook him.'

All of which could be said with equal truth of Dean Buckland.

Although Jenner's grants from Parliament —the cause of much envy and ill-will—amounted to nearly £28,000, he does not appear to have been a rich man. He was evidently free with his

money—offering a thousand pounds towards furnishing a properly-equipped ship in order to
introduce vaccination into India, and, no doubt,
spending a considerable amount on publishing,
correspondence, travelling, charity, and on gifts to
relations.

In a letter to James Moore (July 23, 1813) he
writes :

' I know you fancy that the *cow* has fattened me and
that it is of no use to attempt altering your opinion.   My
state of domestication is the same now as it was before
I cultivated her acquaintance so closely ;   except, that
then I had horses to my carriage, and that *now I have none*. . . .
To know anything about me you should come down and
inquire of my neighbours what I am, and what I was.'

CHAPTER 8

World-wide spread of vaccination. Jenner's charitable work in retirement. As a country magistrate. Visit to Matthew Baillie. Physical and mental depression. Death. Burial in Berkeley Church. Monument in Gloucester Cathedral.

So, from the pleasant Vale of Berkeley, with its meadows and dairy-farms, there had gone forth, while the world was at war, a simple rite—rapidly spreading through all countries, from Iceland and Greenland (where smallpox had in one year slain one-fourth of its people) to Southern China—from the Ural mountains to Mexico and to Indian tribes in North and South America—a rite which had saved the lives of countless human beings, and was destined to save the lives of millions yet unborn. Nothing quite like it had happened in the known history of the world—this sudden arrest of a universal and dreaded pestilence.

Although burdened with correspondence, Jenner found time to attend to the affairs of the 'village,' where he was the only magistrate. The country-side—even the Vale of Berkeley—had lost some of the charm it had possessed when Jenner, with all the health and good spirits of youth, full of schemes for promoting the advancement of medical knowledge, active, and generous, as fond of his neighbours as they were of him, began his rides over the country half a century before.

Taxation, due to the Napoleonic wars, had fallen heavily on the land. The smaller landowners were selling their lands to the large landowners—farmers, after a sudden unhealthy prosperity, were ruined—labourers were poverty-stricken.

So Jenner had other duties besides those of a country doctor. Baron[1] found him one day in a

'dark tobacco-flavoured room listening to parish business of various sorts. The door was surrounded by a scolding, brawling mob. A fat overseer of the poor was endeavouring to moderate their noise. . . . There were women swearing . . . the peace against drunken husbands, and able-bodied men demanding parish relief to make up the deficiency in their wages. . . . He said to me, " Is not this too bad ? I am the only acting magistrate in this place. I want the Lord Lieutenant to give me an assistant ; and I have applied for my nephew, but without success." . . .

' He showed me the hide of the cow, that afforded the matter which infected Sarah Helmes, and from which source he derived virus that produced the disease in Phipps. The hide hung in the coach house.[2] . . . The

[1] Baron : *Life of Jenner*, ii. 303.
[2] It now hangs in the Museum at St. George's Hospital.

cow had been turned out to end her days peaceably at a farm near Berkeley.'

James Phipps, the first vaccinated patient, contracted pulmonary tubercle in later life. Jenner built him a cottage, and, partly with his own hands, planted the garden.

In 1820 he spent some days with the well-known Matthew Baillie at Duntisbourne. Dr. Matthew Baillie—one of the chief physicians of his time, John Hunter's nephew, Physician to St. George's Hospital, Censor of the College of Physicians, and Physician Extraordinary to George III, whom he attended during the King's last illness, 'kind, generous, and sincere' [1]—after refusing a baronetcy had retired to an estate which he had purchased at Duntisbourne, near Cirencester.

Baron says of Baillie :

'It was cheering to see the great London physician mounted on his little white horse, riding up and down precipitous banks, or trotting through the green lanes, and opening the gates, just after the manner of any Cotswold squire. Nothing could exceed the relish of Baillie for the ease, and liberty, and leisure of a country life, when he first escaped from the toil and excitement of his professional duties in London.'

Baillie was among the first to appreciate the value

[1] Sir Henry Halford, in Munk's *Roll of the Royal College of Physicians,* p. 407.

of vaccination and to vindicate its virtue ; and
Jenner, in his walks with him, forgot, for a time,
his sorrow at the loss of his wife and eldest son,
and the attacks of the anti-vaccinists. He delighted
in pointing out to Baillie the country round
Cirencester he knew so well, and the oolite rocks,
in which, as a schoolboy, he had found fossils.

It was a pleasant scene—this fraternising of the
two tired medicos, who had served their generation
well. But it was a scene in the last act of the
drama. Within three years the curtain had been
rung down on both lives.

Jenner was now feeling the effects of the strenu-
ous life on which he had entered when past
middle age. In 1820 he had an attack of uncon-
sciousness, from which, under the care of his
nephew and Henry Shrapnell, he slowly recovered.

He was able to renew his correspondence on the
subject nearest his heart. But noises troubled him,
and he remained over-sensitive to sharp sounds.
In a letter to the Rev. Dr. Worthington (Aug. 2,
1821) he says :

' I have been a fixture in this joyless spot, and here
I am likely to remain till removed in one way or another.
. . . I am as susceptible as you ever saw me to those
pointed sounds emanating from the utensils which spread
over our dinner and breakfast tables—the blunt noises
such as issue from a peal of bells I regard not. I stood

at the foot of the tower (of Berkeley Church) a short time since, and regarded it no more than the hum of Gray's beetle,[1] which now enchants my garden every evening. The cry of hounds would still be music to me ; but the horrible *click* of a spoon, knife, or fork falling upon a plate gives my brain a kind of death blow. You see then that I am almost driven out of society by this misfortune, if one may be allowed to call anything a misfortune which occurs to us during our journey through life.'

In another letter he wrote :

' I boast of my strength in the morning, but evening comes before its time. Such are the workings of the old partners of mind and body after the firm has been very long established. . . . The humble submission to what we are apt to suppose our misfortunes is the best smoother of the rugged roads of life.'

So, with diminishing vitality, and in the loneliness of old age, he continued his work, anxious only that the sacred cause of vaccination should not suffer from unskilled hands, or from the delays brought about by those who, jealous of his success, unfairly attacked it. Occasionally he thought that ' vaccination will go on just as well when I am dead as it does during my existence—probably better, for one obstacle will die with me—envy.' Reports of its failure were worrying him. In a

[1] Gray's *Elegy* : ' The beetle wheels his droning flight.'

letter to his niece, Miss Kingscote (January 10, 1823), he says :

'. . . You are very good in writing so kindly to me after my *seeming* neglect of you all. You think me idle, no doubt, . . . if you did but know the laborious work I have to go through, your opinion would soon be changed . . . at any period of my long life, I do not think there was ever a period when I worked harder. It is no bodily exertion, of course, that I allude to ; but it is that which is far more oppressive, the toils of the mind. I am harassed and oppressed beyond anything you can have a conception of. In the midst of these embarrassments I have not a soul about me who can afford me assistance, except my two good-humoured nieces who copy letters for me, and would willingly do more if they could.'

But he recovered his good spirits, and on January 24, 1823, walked to the village of Ham, in order to arrange a distribution of fuel to the poor. It was cold—the thermometer many degrees below freezing-point — but Jenner accomplished the journey without difficulty. On his return he walked into his nephew Stephen's painting room— detected some inaccuracy in a Scotch air his nephew was singing—and sang two stanzas himself. The following morning, at breakfast time, he was found insensible on the floor of his library. A blood-vessel in the brain had given way ; his right side was paralysed ; he died the next morning.

K

And so passed away one who, against natural inclination, had been compelled to join the ranks of the immortals—a country practitioner who was destined to save more lives than the wars, which raged during his lifetime, had destroyed.

A few days later he was laid to rest beside his wife in the chancel of Berkeley Church.

It is an interesting story—the young countryman, so devoted to a rare bit of the soil of old England that he has no use of the world's honours, or fame, returning—he hopes for life—to his own village, fascinated by the beauty of the country—its valleys and hills, its green lanes and its birds—content and happy in the company of his neighbours : then, in the autumn of life, hearing a call compelling him, though a man of slow speech, to go and preach the good news of vaccination, in all the turmoil of opposition and controversy, to a world from which he had fled.

At a meeting of medical men in Gloucester, it was proposed to erect a monument to Jenner in the Cathedral. Subscriptions were asked for ; but came in slowly. Everyone was poor, except the war profiteers, and they were not inclined to give money so recently acquired. The only public bodies which helped were the Royal College of Physicians of Edinburgh, which generously sent £50, and the Royal College of Surgeons of Edinburgh, which contributed £10. Eventually, enough money was raised to give an order to Sievier for a statue.

In 1858 a bronze statue of Jenner was unveiled by the Prince Consort in Trafalgar Square. It was not the right place. So, just as Jenner himself fled from London to his own countryside, the statue, in four years' time, was transferred to Kensington Gardens. There, amidst more appropriate sur-roundings, Jenner looks down, from a green bank, upon wild ducks and moorhens swimming among water plants at the head of the Long Water.

CHAPTER 9

A FEW years after Jenner's death, Dr. Baron wrote a *Life of Jenner*, full of admiration for Jenner and for his work. Half a century afterwards another book appeared, two heavy volumes,[1] which attempted to prove that Jenner's work was fallacious, and that vaccination ' does not exercise any protective power against human smallpox.'

In the same year a writer of importance, Charles Creighton, M.D., wrote a book of three hundred pages [2]—a passionate attack on Jenner and vaccination. Creighton had studied in Berlin and Vienna, and had attempted practice in London— without success. There was in his nature some

---

[1] *History of Vaccination*, by E. M. Crookshank, Professor of Comparative Pathology, King's College, 1889, i. 464.

[2] C. Creighton : *Jenner and Vaccination. A Strange Chapter in Medical History*, 1889. The book is not to be found in the College of Physicians or College of Surgeons libraries.

curious flaw, which kept him out of touch with fellow-men. His days were spent in working alone in the British Museum and other libraries. Professor W. Bulloch, in an obituary notice,[1] says of Creighton, ' He was a scholar and philosopher . . . the most learned man I ever knew. . . . He spoke and read nearly all the European languages . . . his *History of Epidemics* [2] is the greatest work of medical learning published in the nineteenth century by an Englishman.' It is ' written with insight and literary brilliance.'

Creighton ' exhibited indifference to the most hostile criticism, and bore no grudge,' but he was roused to fury by Baron's admiration of Jenner.

It is not always kind to bestow too much praise on a friend. Although some hear with pleasure what seems to be excessive praise given to a fellow-creature—reminding them of the lovableness hidden in ordinary human nature—others seem to be roused by it to fierce hostility, and a longing to find out, and proclaim to all the world, the hero's weaknesses. Creighton was one of the latter.

Creighton [3] begins by attacking Jenner for his paper on the young cuckoo, which he considers a deliberate lie. The ' unique and marvellous

---

[1] W. Bulloch : *Lancet,* July 30, 1927 ; *Aberdeen University Review,* March 1928.

[2] C. Creighton : *History of Epidemics in Great Britain,* 1891.

[3] C. Creighton : *Jenner and Vaccination,* 1889, p. 17.

structural change' of the back, he writes, 'it need hardly be said, has no existence . . . the greater part of the paper, and all that part of it which is best remembered, is a tissue of inconsistencies and absurdities.'

Having thus prepared the ground for his attack on Jenner's more important work, Creighton, who had ransacked journals both at home and abroad in quest of anything that would tell against Jenner and vaccination, makes an unwarranted attack on Jenner himself, as an impostor, deliberately intending to mislead the public, especially in his term for cow-pox, '*variolæ vaccinæ*'—'smallpox of the cow,' without any scientific evidence that it was. Creighton declares that the medical profession in all countries 'fell under the enchantment of an illusion' misled by the title of Jenner's pamphlet. He continues : 'of the many sly and impudent tales that Jenner told to the medical profession, and to the public, this is the most sly, and the most impudent.'[1] Creighton's onslaught suggests the lawyer's indictment of Mr. Pickwick, for his 'overt, sly, communications.'

Creighton was a master of English. Jenner found difficulty in expressing his ideas, and perhaps failed in stating his case as logically as Creighton would have done. Words, even those of the wisest,

---

[1] C. Creighton : *Jenner and Vaccination*, 1889, p. 163.

are but imperfect means of conveying thought—
in fact they often obscure it—but Jenner's observations, and the mental deductions which he made
from them, but was unable to state fully on paper,
proved to be true. Just as his account of the
extraordinary acts of the young cuckoo have been
shown to be accurate, and Creighton's accusations
unjustified, so the statement that cow-pox is smallpox transmitted through the cow has now been
proved to be correct, by successfully inoculating
calves with the virus of *inoculated* smallpox,[1] and so
producing vaccine lymph. Creighton's attack on
Jenner was an instance—not a solitary one—of
profound, learned, logical, statistical conclusions
being wrong, and those of observant, thoughtful
common sense being right.

The centenary of Jenner's death was celebrated
at the *Académie de Médecine* in Paris in January
1923, and honour was done to Jenner's memory.
(Why are deathdays of great men celebrated rather
than their birthdays?) Professor Tessier gave an
address on Jenner. He pointed out in eloquent
words that in the short Franco-German war of
1870–1, with few men engaged—most of them
unvaccinated—there were nearly 30,000 deaths
from smallpox; whereas in the Great War, among

[1] See *Vaccination*, by S. Monckton Copeman, M.D., F.R.S., 1899.

4,000,000 men, carefully vaccinated or revaccinated, there were only four cases.[1]

At the same time, a special meeting of the Royal Society of Medicine was held in London, in honour of Jenner. It was presided over by Sir William Hale-White, who gave a sketch of Jenner's life and character. ' Jenner,' he said, ' freely gave of that most valuable of all commodities —his time—he would listen to all callers, rich or poor.'

At this meeting members, as they came to the door, were plentifully supplied with anti-vaccination pamphlets—the prophet, as usual, finding his chief opponents in his own country.

The obvious, spectacular success of vaccination in Jenner's day may have been partly due to the fact that lymph was obtained directly from cows which had been accidentally inoculated with smallpox by milkers. In an interesting letter, written to Jenner from Cambridge, U.S.A., on April 24, 1801, Dr. Waterhouse says :

' At one of our periodical inoculations, which occur once in . eight years, several persons drove their cows to an hospital near a village, in order that their families might have the benefit of their milk. These cows were milked by persons in all stages of the smallpox. The consequence was the cows had an eruptive disorder so

---

[1] *British Medical Journal*, February 3, 1923.

like the smallpox pustule that everyone in the hospital declared the cows had smallpox.'

It has been proved that cows are far more susceptible to virus from the vesicles of inoculated smallpox than to virus from casual smallpox contracted in the usual way.

This points to the interesting conclusion that if inoculation for smallpox had not been introduced into England there would have been no cow-pox, and consequently no vaccination. Sarah Nelmes would not have had the historic vesicle on her hand if the cow she milked had not been milked the week before by someone recovering from smallpox *inoculation*.

A century and a half of vaccination has now almost banished smallpox from countries in which vaccination has been efficient, and has reduced it, when it does occur, to what is often a mild illness—so mild that it occasionally escapes recognition. Not only does the eruption of smallpox vary greatly both in appearance and intensity, but the strains of vaccine lymph vary, and vaccinators themselves vary, as they did in Jenner's day ; and up to more recent times, when—as an authority relates—it was possible to earn a precarious living somewhere on the West Coast of Africa by ' vaccinating with condensed milk at half a crown a head.' So some failures there have been, and must be, and no statistics of any kind can be perfectly truthful,[1] but the overwhelming testimony of all nations, in Jenner's time, to the arrest of a dreaded, universal, curse of humanity, ought to be sufficient evidence to convince those who doubt the efficacy of vaccination, and the priceless boon it was to the world.

Those of us who, as revaccinated doctors, students, or nurses, moved with impunity among smallpox patients during the epidemics of 1878 and 1884 require no convincing.

In 1889 a Royal Commission was appointed to enquire into the results of vaccination. It reported in 1896 that vaccination diminished the liability to an attack of smallpox, that in proportion to the number of those who underwent vaccination the number of those who suffered in any way from it was insignificant, and also that repeated penalties for non-vaccination should no longer be enforced.

A minority report recommended that compulsory vaccination should be abolished altogether.[2]

---

[1] Sir Almroth Wright, M.D., F.R.S., gave a warning on statistics when speaking on a paper on 'Vaccination' read by Professor Greenwood, F.R.S., at a meeting of the Statistical Society when he said, ' Statistical methods are not applicable to investigations into the efficiency of particular ways of dealing with disease. The statistician demanded large figures. The attempts to obtain them were liable to assemble facts which were dissimilar. The facts which impressed him were isolated cases where cause and effect were definitely proved.' *Royal Statistical Society Journal*, vol. xciii. pt. 2, 1930.

[2] Sir William Collins, M.P., in the House of Commons debate, February 15, 1907.

In two years' time an amended vaccination Act allowed conscientious objectors to have their way. This was followed by a great falling off in infantile vaccinations.

Among the poor vaccination has always been unpopular. Its present discomfort is always more apparent than its ultimate advantage. The Sunday school child who, in reply to a question why Moses was hidden in the bulrushes, said ' Because they wanted to vaccinate him,' gave what he thought a very good reason.

In a preface to the Minority Report of the Royal Commission of 1896, Sir William Collins writes :

' This falling off in vaccination has not only been un-accompanied by any increased mortality from smallpox, but the disease that has been prevalent of late has been remarkably mild in character and of exceptionally low fatality.'

There is now in England so complete a system for notification and isolation of infectious cases under vigilant sanitary authorities, that, except for those who have just been, or are likely to be, exposed to infection, the need for vaccination is far less than it was in Jenner's day. But the need remains as before among those who are about to be exposed to infection.

During the epidemic of 1902, the late D. L. Thomas reported that twenty-four efficiently re-vaccinated members of a staff of thirty-one at the Mile End Infirmary escaped smallpox, but that *all* the unprotected ones—seven in number—contracted it.

A commission appointed by the League of Nations collected information on the whole subject of vaccination, and in a Government Report[1] of 1930, Dr. F. R. Blaxall writes : ' It is recognised in all civilised countries that vaccination and re-vaccination afford a sure protection against small-pox,'[2] and that during and after the war small-pox spread rapidly in such countries as Russia, Italy, and Roumania, ' where vaccination pre-cautions were necessarily relaxed.'[3]

Dr. Blaxall states the interesting fact that al-though smallpox in the cow is transmuted into cow-pox, in monkeys it is not—that during an epidemic among natives in Brazil many dead monkeys with a typical smallpox eruption were found under the trees.

Unfortunately of late years, an inflammation of the brain has occasionally followed vaccination, as it has measles and other illnesses ; so, in England,

---

[1] *System of Bacteriology*, vii. 124, an exhaustive and erudite report on vaccination—73 pages quarto—published by the Privy Council, 1930.
[2] *Ibid.* 124.   [3] *Ibid.* 87.

vaccination is now carried out at one spot only in the patient's arm—repeated before school age—and again later.[1]

The Report states that the vaccine now used in England is derived from a strain of calf lymph received from Cologne in 1907, and maintained with most careful precautions (antiseptic and otherwise) by passage from calf to calf, or more readily, through young rabbits. It is diluted with glycerine, which—as Copeman pointed out—slowly destroys any unwelcome germs. It is then put away in cold storage for many months before it is considered ready for use.[2]

Jenner vaccinated with lymph obtained from horses and cows ; he could not have dreamed that it would one day be obtained from rabbits !

[1] Vaccination Order, 1929.   [2] *System of Bacteriology*, vii. 121.

INDEX

Printed in England at THE BALLANTYNE PRESS
SPOTTISWOODE, BALLANTYNE & CO. LTD.
Colchester, London & Eton